FIND THE
ROOT CAUSE
OF YOUR ANXIETY

BEAT ANXIETY FOR *GOOD!*

MICHELE PENCE, H.C.

© Michele Pence 2014

All rights reserved. No part of this publication may be reproduced, distributed, or transmitted in any form or by any means, including photocopying, recording, or other electronic or mechanical methods, without the prior written permission, except in the case of brief quotations embodied in critical reviews and certain other noncommercial uses permitted under copyright law.

This book is not intended as a substitute for the medical advice of physicians. The reader should regularly consult a physician in matters relating to his/her health and particularly with respect to any symptoms that may require diagnosis and medical attention.

Cover by: Steven James Catizone

For my husband, Byron, and our two amazing sons, Julian and Noah.

Thank you for standing by me every step of the way!

Table of Contents

FORWARD .... **III**
INTRODUCTION .... **V**
CHAPTER 1 WHAT IS ANXIETY? **1**
    ANXIETY VS. STRESS 2
    UNDERSTANDING STRESS 3
    HOW IS ANXIETY DIFFERENT? 4
    DO I SUFFER FROM ANXIETY? 4
    COMMON SIGNS AND SYMPTOMS OF ANXIETY 7
    TYPES OF ANXIETY 8
    DIAGNOSIS AND TREATMENT 12
CHAPTER 2 HOW HORMONES AFFECT YOUR BODY **17**
    WHERE DO HORMONES COME FROM? 18
    KNOW YOUR HORMONES 37
    BALANCE IN ALL THINGS 42
CHAPTER 3 UNDERSTANDING NEUROTRANSMITTERS **47**
    NEUROTRANSMITTERS AND ANXIETY 48
    CALMING YOUR INTERNAL FAMILY 54
CHAPTER 4 TOXINS IN OUR MISTS **57**
    BENZENE 58
    BPA 59
    FORMALDEHYDE POISONING 60
    MERCURY & HEAVY METAL 61
    MAXIMIZE YOUR SAFETY AROUND TOXINS 68
CHAPTER 5 DIET & EXERCISE **71**
    INCORPORATING EXERCISE INTO THERAPY 72
    YOUR DIET AND ANXIETY 74
    BALANCED NUTRITION AND EXERCISE 81
CHAPTER 6 ADDICTION & DEPENDENCY **85**
    ALCOHOL 86
    CAFFEINE 89
    FOOD ADDICTION 90
    ILLEGAL DRUGS 97
    MARIJUANA 97
    PRESCRIPTION MEDICATION 98
    TOBACCO 102

DEPENDENCY AND EMOTIONAL WELL-BEING 102
CHAPTER 7 ALLERGENS & THE ENVIRONMENT 107
   FOOD ALLERGENS 108
   INDOOR HOUSEHOLD ALLERGENS... 114
   KNOW YOUR TRIGGERS 116
CHAPTER 8 COMMON HEALTH CONDITIONS 119
   ANEMIA 119
   ASTHMA 120
   DIABETES 121
   INSOMNIA 125
   LUPUS 127
   MENOPAUSE 128
   MTHFR GENE MUTATION 128
CHAPTER 9 TRACKING THE ROOT CAUSE 131
   REQUIRED TESTS 132
   SUGGESTED TESTS 135
CHAPTER 10 NATURAL TREATMENT OPTIONS 137
   COMBAT THE PROBLEM HEAD ON 138
   CREATE A MANTRA 139
   MEDITATE 140
   DON'T FORGET YOUR SUPPORT GROUP 141
   SWEAT AWAY ANXIETY 144
   EAT A HEALTHY DIET 144
   GET PLENTY OF SLEEP 145
   ORGANIZE 146
   FORGET THE JONESES!! 147
   SET GOALS FOR YOURSELF 149
   SUPPLEMENTS 150
   BEATING ANXIETY FOR GOOD! 150
INDEX 153
RESOURCES & REFERENCES 157
ABOUT THE AUTHOR 159

Forward

Michele is a courageous woman who arrived at my office willing to do whatever it takes to feel well again. It has been a joy to work with her and to watch her gain insight into the root cause of her anxiety, fatigue and general disease. She has helped to raise my awareness of the implications of a 5-MTHFR alteration and the many people who suffer the consequences.

Understanding YOUR biochemistry is the key to understanding the root cause of your ailments and challenges. Michele is an example of someone who takes charge of their wellness and digs deep to find the answers. It is not easy to do what she has done. I wish all my patients would take such ownership. Let her story empower you to act, seek and choose wellness.

Lisbeth W Roy, DO.
Chief Medical Officer

Introduction

You may be wondering why I would choose to write a book about anxiety. And, why I'd choose such a bold title as Find the Root Cause of YOUR Anxiety: Beat Anxiety for Good! After all, countless doctors and psychiatrists have already expounded on the topic in numerous scholarly journals.

The answer is simple. I've been there. I know what it's like to wake up in the middle of the night in a cold sweat, terrified about the circumstances around me. I've fought with the demons of hopelessness at feeling totally out of control in a situation. I've struggled to take action when I knew failure was imminent. And I've cycled the medication merry-go-round in search of a wonder cure for these symptoms.

Chances are if you're reading this book, you or someone you know has gone through that same cycle of anxiety and hopelessness only to seek refuge in a medicine bottle. Your doctor may even tell you that's your only option for treatment.

That's what mine told me.

For almost fifteen years, I was convinced that my only hope for combating my anxiety issues was through medication. Unfortunately, when medication is the only answer, your body can become dependent to it and immune to its effects. The longer I took it, the less it seemed to work. I needed more to feel the same level of comfort and soon after that, more still. It became a dangerous cycle for me until one day in 2012 when I made the decision to find the root cause for my condition and combat those issues instead.

It's been a long hard journey for me. If you've been taking medication for anxiety for a significant amount of time, it will be for you as well. But I was able to successfully complete my goal to be medication free since 2013 with the help of good friends, a supportive family, forward thinking doctors, and my faith. What I learned during that process is that anxiety, like so many other conditions, is a disease in its own right, but it is also a symptom of numerous other conditions and circumstances. It may have just as much to do with the environmental conditions at your work as it does with an overactive thyroid gland. It may be a sign of a far worse medical condition such as diabetes or a heart condition. Or, it may be a side effect of medication such as albuterol or methyldopa. There are hundreds of contributing factors that when combined together can cause anxiety.

The great news is – if you truly want to fight your anxiety issues and reduce medication intake, you can. I was able to completely eliminate anti-anxiety medication from my system and you can too. By learning the underlying causes that trigger anxiety, you can modify your life to purge anxiety medication from your life. In doing so, you can alleviate many of the symptoms of anxiety that often cripple your success and your productivity.

In the pages of this book you will find a wealth of information about anxiety and its many cases. You will begin to see the relationship before body chemistry, hormonal harmony, and personal well being that will enhance your life like never before. You will discover the environmental and external factors that contribute to your anxiousness. And you will learn how to confront these issues head on and win your personal battle with anxiety.

Now, before we begin our journey toward an anxiety free lifestyle, I must strongly advise you NOT to stop taking any medications you are currently using without first consulting your personal physician. I am not advocating the cold turkey approach. I know from experience (as you will see later on) that approach doesn't work.

On the contrary, I recommend you to work with your doctor to determine if there are other causes for your anxiety that you haven't considered. Then, if you are able, consider working with them to safely wean your body off these types of medications. If your doctor won't work with you on this, find a new doctor who will. I suggest you to incorporate an improved diet and exercise routine that wards off the demons of the past. And I want you to grow stronger each day in the knowledge that you are actively improving your life and the lives of all those around you.

Once your body is free from the leash of anxiety medication, you will begin to feel a sense of calm and relief you never knew existed. I'm excited that you've chosen to take this journey with me. I have full confidence that you will be as successful in your voyage as I have been on mine, if not more so. I know you can feel better than you ever dreamt possible.

Chapter 1 What Is Anxiety?

According to the Anxiety and Depression Association of America, anxiety is the most common mental illness in America today. It affects over 40 million adults over the age of 18. That equals over 18% of the U.S. population.

Think about that for a moment. That is almost the entire population of Spain!! Or to put it another way, it's the combined population of Portugal, Greece, Belgium, and Switzerland. To put it mildly, that is a lot of people.

In terms of financial losses, anxiety disorders cost the United States over $42 billion per year. (That's billion with a capital B!) In fact, about 1/3 of this country's annual mental health expenditures are directly related to anxiety disorders. Patients who suffer from anxiety are four times more likely to seek medical treatment for ailments and pain, especially back pain and headaches than non sufferers. And they are six times more likely to be admitted to the hospital for other mental disorders than non sufferers. Women make up almost 2/3 of the anxiety patients.

The same does not seem to hold true in Europe. For example, it is estimated that in the United Kingdom less than 900 thousand adults suffer from Generalized Anxiety Disorder, a tiny fraction of the more than 60 billion citizens. France presents almost a mirror image of the statistics in the UK. Only Germany exceeds a million, with 1.2 million adults estimated to suffer from General Anxiety Disorder. Even that is a small percentage of their 82+ billion populace.

DID YOU KNOW?

Jean Arthur, the famous 1930s and 1940s starlit of such films as "Mr. Smith Goes to Washington" and "Only Angels Have Wings," was so stricken with anxiety and panic attacks prior to a scene that she would often spend hours in her dressing too physically ill to perform. She eventually retired from cinema in 1944 despite her growing popularity with the general public.

Before we begin our journey into the root causes of anxiety, it is important to fully understand what anxiety actually is and what it is not. All too often, people confuse anxiety disorders with day-to-day stress. Sometimes, people are over treated for conditions they do not have. Unfortunately, the reverse is more often true. Those who need help the most rarely seek help because they assume what they feel is normal.

Anxiety vs. Stress

We all have things in our lives that cause tension and stress. It may not be the most enjoyable part of life but it's normal. There is little we can do to alleviate all the stress from our lives. So how can we tell if the nervousness we're feeling is merely because of day-to-day stress or something more complex, like full blown anxiety?

Understanding Stress

Stress can most easily be defined as your reaction to a particular event or situation in your life. It may trigger the fight or flight response in which you may or may not want to run into the safest corner. It can cause sleepless nights, fatigue, and a loss of appetite. But it will only last for the duration of the situation you're in.

Take a CPA for example. Each spring her calendar is filled to capacity with businesses and individuals in need of tax preparation services. She knows this in advance and schedules her time accordingly. Even still, with too many clients to manage and too few hours in the day, this period of time is extremely stressful. She may be losing sleep not only because of the added stress of her workload but because she is staying up until midnight each night working on returns for clients. However, on April 16th of each year, that burden disappears almost immediately. There will still be a few clients who need tax preparation and accounting services. She will still be busy throughout the year, but the immediate, overwhelming stress is gone until next year at the same time.

Typically, if asked, you can pinpoint the specific condition which is causing your tension although there are some cases where this may not be the case. It is possible to live in a stressful situation so long that you actually forget the toll stress is taking on your body. For example, if you are the long term care giver for a parent with Alzheimer's disease and you have cared for her for a year or more, you may have adjusted to the level of stress you are constantly under although that stress is still taking a physical toll on your body. You will feel more fatigued than before, perhaps more agitated, and moody. You may gain weight and become irritable. These are all common signs and symptoms of stress that you did not have before and, theoretically, wouldn't have after your stress was removed.

How Is Anxiety Different?

On the other hand, anxiety is a monster unto its own. While some of the signs and symptoms of anxiety may be the same as those of stress, the two are drastically different.

Anxiety does not need a specific catalyst. (Don't confuse catalyst with root cause! There are root causes that can trigger anxiety issues which we'll discuss in detail in Chapters 2-9!) When we speak about a catalyst in this context, we are referring to a specific event or occurrence that triggers an anxiety episode.

Let's look back at our CPA. She had a specific event that triggered her stress – the tax preparation season. However, if she had difficulty functioning at work, if she panicked with each accounting entry she made for clients throughout the year, or if she couldn't bring herself to get out of bed and go to work each day because of an overwhelming and irrational fear, then she may be suffering from anxiety in some form.

Do I Suffer From Anxiety?

Below is a simple test which will help determine if you are a victim of anxiety in some form or other. Beside each corresponding symptom, annotate the frequency of the occurrence using numbers 1 through 5 with 1 being never and 5 meaning usually.

Signs and Symptoms	Never 1	Rarely 2	Sometimes 3	Often 4	Usually 5
Heart feels like it will jump out of your chest					
Prolonged or unusual sweating					
Hands and feet tremble					
Difficulty catching your breath					
Feelings of fear					
Pain and tightness in the chest					
Bloated or irritable bowels					
Feeling light headed					
Worry that you're losing control of a situation					
Numbness in the hands and feet					
Seek to avoid uncomfortable situations					
Feel as though you may faint					

Random, unexplained twitches					
Loss of sleep					
Feel unsteady or off balance					
Have constant nervous feeling					
Unable to wind down					
Constant feeling of worry					
Fear of death					
Feel as though nothing in life is real					

Add up your answers on a separate sheet of paper. If you scored 0-5, congratulations! Your life is virtually stress free. The rest of us envy you greatly! Likewise if you received a score of 6-19, you lead a relatively calm and collected life. You have some stress but you have managed it well. However, if you scored between 20-34, you are dealing with a fairly persistent level of anxiety. You will want to explore your options for life style modifications or contact your physician to uncover the root causes for your condition. For a score over 35, you are suffering from extreme anxiety. You know your life isn't fun right now but you have no idea how to make it better or where to even begin.

Common Signs and Symptoms of Anxiety

As we will learn in the next section there are several different types of anxiety which manifest in different ways. While each patient is distinctive and each case unique, there are some common signs and symptoms that are routinely experienced on a regular basis.

- Uneasiness and fear: For some people this can be an overwhelming sensation of panic for no apparent reason. For others, it is a never-ending feeling of doom or dread.
- Sleep disruption: Unlike patients who suffer exclusively from depression, sufferers of anxiety will often face long bouts where they are unable to go to sleep. They may suddenly wake in the middle of the night unable to return to sleep. Often these individuals become so exhausted that they eventually crash and sleep for an extended period of time.
- Breathing difficulties: Some patients have likened this to a brick wall or elephant sitting on their chest, making if physically impossible to breathe.
- Fidgetiness: Patients may pace or twitch without the slightest idea they are moving. Even while sitting their knees or hands will be in constant motion.
- Nausea and irregular bowel activities: When experiencing an attack, many patients will become ill at the mere thought of food. They may forget to eat. They often suffer from Irritable Bowel Syndrome.
- Heart flutters: Also known as palpitations, these episodes may seem like a heart attack to the person

experiencing them. Some have said, "it feels like your heart is trying to jump out of your chest."

Types of Anxiety

Now that we understand the basic difference between day-to-day stress and anxiety, we need to take a look at the different types of anxiety people commonly suffer from. There are four main categories of anxiety conditions. As you will see, there are varying degrees of severity with each condition. You will also find that many of these conditions have overlapping signs and symptoms. For example, a person may suffer from Generalized Anxiety Disorder but experience a phobia of snakes. This overlapping is not uncommon, however it is vital to fully understand what type of anxiety you suffer from and what potential triggers may aggravate your anxiety symptoms.

Generalized Anxiety Disorder

This is the most common diagnosis among anxiety sufferers as it is the least likely to have a specific external cause. Women are twice as likely to be diagnosed with GAD as men. Sufferers constantly worry about multiple aspects of their lives including trivia or mundane issues. They live in constant fear that they do not 'measure up' or have failed in some way.

For the vast majority of patients, GAD symptoms begin in adolescence or early adulthood, although symptoms may manifest at any time. They may worry about a particular project for school or work in excess, with the most severe cases causing a failure to perform under pressure. Sufferers may find it difficult to concentrate; may experience headaches, fatigue, and abdominal irritability; may have difficulty sleeping and be unable to relax for even the briefest periods of time; or they may suffer from frequent sweating or hot flashes.

In some cases, GAD will be diagnosed with other conditions such as Post Traumatic Stress Disorder, Social Anxiety Disorder, or Obsessive Compulsive Disorder.

Panic Disorder

It is estimated that Panic Disorder affects 2.4 million Americans over the age of 18. This anxiety disorder may be present in conjunction with GAD or several other types of anxiety disorders, however, it, in and of itself, can cause anxiety within the patient.

Sufferers from Panic Disorder experience severe episodes of panic induced fear known as panic attacks. These attacks will generally last for 10 minutes or more. During this event, patients may display signs and symptoms similar to a heart attack including chest pains, difficulty breathing, nausea, and sweating. They may feel that death is imminent. Additionally, they may experience numbness, chills or hot flashes, and overwhelming sensation of smothering. Some have likened the experience to an elephant sitting on their chest.

Once the patient has experienced a panic attack, they then develop a fear of future panic attacks. They may feel a complete loss of control over their emotional and physical wellbeing. They live in constant stress that another attack may happen at any moment. Therein lies the main factor with this condition, anxiety itself causes anxiety. It is this constant worry which causes suffers the greatest level of anxiety.

Phobias

Phobia is defined as 'anxiety brought on by a specific event or object.' All of us have a fear of something. Whether you fear snakes, clowns, crowds, or heights, we all have things that will instantly trigger fear.

In the vast majority of situations, when we encounter such an object, we pause to evaluate the situation thoroughly before determining the best course of action. Perhaps we have a fear of flying but are required by our job to travel extensively. We may bring a good book to read or soothing music to calm our nerves. We may exercise before the flight to release negative tension. We may develop a ritual for each flight that we follow to help ease the tension. However, we face that uneasy feeling and adjust to the situation at hand.

A phobia, however, is more extreme than just a simple fear. Phobia suffers may seek out ways to avoid the situation or object which triggers the fear regardless of the inconvenience this avoidance may cause. In the example above, a person with a severe phobia of flying might avoid flying all together, choosing other forms of transportation. This choice could cause that patient to spend less time with family and friends, increase the overall expense of the travel, or cause the patient to lose the job in question.

Unlike other forms of anxiety, phobias have a specific external trigger. However, similar to other conditions, the level of anxiety caused by the trigger may be dependent on many factors as we'll see in later chapters.

Social Anxiety Disorder

When most people hear the term social anxiety disorder, they tend to think of a fear of crowds. While this may be a symptom of the condition, SAD is much more complex. People who suffer from social anxiety disorder have an intense fear of ridicule and embarrassment. The thought of being judged by others is paralyzing to them.

Many of us have felt a tinge of nervousness at the thought of giving a speech to a large group of people or of going to an important job interview. These are normal stressors which we overcome and adapt to. However, individuals with SAD may have difficulties leaving home or interacting with others around them in any type of social setting. They may worry for days or weeks about an upcoming event or they may avoid social events all together. Often times this fear is compounded by a person's inability to effectively communicate with others. They may come across as awkward and shy.

Perhaps the best, and most extreme, example many of us have for this condition comes from the popular TV comedy hit, The Big Bang Theory. For many seasons, Dr. Rajesh Koothrappali struggled to make even the most rudimentary sounds when in the presence of a woman. Granted this is an excessive case exaggerated for the purposes of television comedy but it does give viewers a glimpse into the complexities of the condition.

Selective mutism is exceptionally rare. However, sufferers may commonly experience anxiety or panic attacks if they find themselves the center of attention in a group of people, forced into social gatherings such as parties or dining out, or working in a public group. Additionally, sufferers from social anxiety may find it difficult to write in front of others or speak on the telephone.

Diagnosis and Treatment

Unfortunately, there is no magic test to diagnose an anxiety condition. There is not one scan that your doctor can perform which will effectively determine the level or type of anxiety you suffer from. A diagnosis will generally be made after a psychological evaluation by a mental health professional. This evaluation is subjective based on question and answer sessions between you and your doctor. Rarely will a complete physical be done to determine if underlying medical, physiological, or hormonal issues exist.

Likewise, the treatment options you are given will be subjective based solely on the experience of your doctor and the evaluation performed. Typically, patients who suffer from anxiety disorders will be prescribed a Benzodiazepine medication such as Xanax or Valium. While these medications may offer immediate relief from the anxiety condition, they do little if anything at all to treat the underlying conditions which cause the vast majority of anxiety symptoms.

Unfortunately, there have been cases where drug companies have offered financial encouragement for physicians who choose their medications over the competition. I will not be addressing those ethical concerns here nor will I assume that any physician you encounter is receiving any type of financial kickback from a pharmaceutical company. I merely want you to be aware that the vast majority of anxiety diagnoses in this country are subjective and made without any concrete data. As such, you, as the patient, must be cautious.

This is why it is critical to fully understand the anxiety diagnosis you have been given and the underlying conditions which may aggravate that condition. You need to take responsibility for your mental, as well as physical, wellbeing to overcome the anxiety you currently feel. You must ensure that your doctor is thoroughly evaluating your entire health picture and not merely writing a prescription to treat the symptom of another condition.

It is your body, your mind, and your life. Take control now and get your life back. Always remember, you deserve to lead a happy life. Don't let anxiety take that happiness away from you.

My Journey into Anxiety

My battle with anxiety began at an early age. I was diagnosed with Attention Deficit Hyperactivity Disorder during the 3rd grade. As such, my doctor prescribed Ritalin to treat the disorder. At that time, the medication was administered only on weekdays during the school year. During holidays, breaks, and on the weekends, I took no medication. For five years, I stayed on Ritalin as my doctor believed by the 8th grade I should have learned to control my overactive mind and sit quietly in class. (I'll discuss the long term effects of Ritalin in Chapter 6!)

As the eldest child, I often worried and worked hard to protect my mother and siblings especially when things got stressful at home. Although, my mother was a rock and held the family together in many ways, I still worried about those around me.

It wasn't until I broke away from an abusive relationship and went off to college that I began to experience difficulty in sleeping and found it difficult to cope with the hurt I felt from my past relationship. So I sought the help of a Psychiatrist, bad mistake. After my first appointment with him he decided to put me on (I was 19 at the time) Effexor (an antidepressant) and he prescribed me Xanax to help me sleep because one of the side effects of Effexor is difficulty in sleeping.

Being young and somewhat naïve about the effects medication can have on the body, I accepted the prescriptions without a moment's hesitation. After all, doctors are trained professionals who know what they're talking about. Why question the judgment of a professional?

Although I only took the Effexor for a short time, I remained on Xanax for over a decade. During that time my Xanax dosage was increased from .25mg per day to 1.5mg per day. You see my body was forming a dependency on anti-anxiety medication to function and that's why I continually needed more for the same affect.

But I didn't realize all this until I started researching benzos and the negative affects they can have on the patients that take them. So in 2012 I started my journey to come off of them. The eventual detoxification process was gut wrenching to say the least. (I'll also speak more about that in Chapter 6!) During that time, I began to notice that the medication I routinely took to alleviate my anxiety actually increased the anxiety I felt. What I didn't know at the time was that there were underlying conditions that were attributing to the cause of the anxiety I felt. Yes, the initial anxiety and lack of sleep was directly caused by moving away from home and dealing with the hurt from an abusive relationship, yet while that caused me great amounts of stress, it was not wholly responsible for the way my body felt. I had to embark on a journey to discover the root cause and heal my body from within.

FIND THE ROOT CAUSE OF YOUR ANXIETY

Chapter 2 How Hormones Affect Your Body

Your body is composed of millions upon millions of cells each working together to operate effectively. Among those cells are hormones. They journey throughout the body through the circulatory system sending messages which determine all major functions your body will perform. Functions such as sexual desire, appetite, mood, and sleep are directly affected by your hormonal levels.

Think of your body as a giant virtual chat room with dozens of participants. One hormone which regulates hunger is talking to another hormone which regulates the production of gastric enzymes. If these two aren't communicating effectively, you will either feel the need to overeat or your body will produce too many enzymes causing an uneasy stomach. Now imagine if this conversation is interrupted because the hormone which regulates mood is overactive and screaming for attention. What should be a systematic free flowing conversation quickly dissolves into an unruly kindergarten class with each individual hormone demanding the most attention.

Needless to say, your body simply can't function effectively like that. If one or two hormones are out of balance, your entire body is out of balance. And, despite what you might think, it only takes small changes in hormone levels to greatly impact everything around you. Have you ever been walking down the street and realized there is a stone in your shoe? When you take the shoe off, you discover it's only a small pebble whereas while you were walking it felt like a huge rock. The same is true of hormone imbalances – the tiniest pebble can rock your entire body!

And most surprisingly, there doesn't have to be an imbalance with your mood controlling hormones to trigger an anxiety attack. Those hormones may be working diligently to control anxiety but the other hormones that interact with them are out of balance. When this happens, your body may begin to experience anxiety or depression as a direct result. You may feel tired and sluggish for no apparent reason. You may have difficulty concentrating. When these symptoms occur, your endocrine system will begin to respond accordingly by increasing or decreasing hormones to counteract the condition. Your body's reaction to other hormone imbalances not normally associated with anxiety may actually cause your anxiety to increase.

I discovered the importance of a harmonious endocrine system when some blood work showed that I had low progesterone, testosterone, and DHEA. This same blood work showed that thyroid levels were not where they should be. He suggested I begin thyroid medication. Against my doctor's advice, I sought out the opinion of a second doctor who began to work with me to uncover the exact cause of my hormonal issues. For me, the thyroid medication would not have been an effective solution because it would not have addressed the true cause of my hormonal imbalances. Once I began to delve deeper into hormones and the endocrine system, I quickly learned that hormones are a science into their own.

Where Do Hormones Come From?

Hormones are produced in a system of glands known as the Endocrine Glands. Derived from the Greek ('endo' meaning within and 'crinis' meaning secrete), the endocrine system comprises eight major glands which produce and secrete hormones directly into the blood stream to be carried throughout the body. These major glands are the thyroid, thymus, hypothalamus, pituitary, pineal, pancreas, adrenal, and the reproductive glands of either the testes or the ovaries. Unlike other glands in the body such as salivary or sweat glands, all the glands in the endocrine system are vascular glands.

Your endocrine system uses feedback to ensure all your body functions are working properly. Think about your home's thermostat for a moment. It regulates the temperature of the air in your home to provide a steady, comfortable temperature for you and your family. Initially, it initiates your HVAC system to send out cooler or warmer air depending on the season of the year. It then receives feedback to determine the overall temperature of the home. Once it receives feedback that the ideal temperature has been reached, it shuts off until the temperature falls out of range of the ideal, at which time the cycle will begin again.

The same is true of your endocrine system. It produces and sends out hormones to regulate appetite, mood, sexual desire, and a host of other bodily responses. Once it receives feedback that the desired ideal has been reached, it will regulate itself to stop sending signals for that particular an activity. A good example is the hormones to control appetite. Your body will tell you when you're hungry and will tell you when you've had enough to eat. Now imagine for a second that there was a miscommunication within this system. If your body does not receive the correct feedback, you continuously feel hungry causing you to overeat. When there is a disconnection within the endocrine system, it's like having a broken thermostat in your home. Your system will keep running and running, all the while sending out incorrect signals for your body.

Thyroid

No other gland or organ in the body is more important in controlling mood than your thyroid. Located in the throat in front of the trachea, this butterfly shaped gland which produces two major hormones – thyroxine and triiodothyonine. They may be difficult to pronounce but they are vital to every aspect of your body. They regulate how your body absorbs or processes fats, your heart rate, body temperature, and the production of protein. Furthermore, every cell in your body needs these thyroid hormones and vitamin D. Cells cannot function properly without it. That's how critical an optimally performing thyroid is to your body.

Did You Know?

Approximately 100 years ago, before the explosion of modern psychiatry, the more accurate and in depth descriptions of clinical depression were found within the pages of textbooks dealing with thyroid disorders. This may be primarily due to the drastic changes in the body when the thyroid fails to function properly. However, that view fell out of favor within the psychiatric community over the years. Even today, many will say it's a case of the chicken versus the egg. Are thyroid issues causing psychiatric problems or are psychiatric problems causing thyroid malfunctions? That debate aside, there is overwhelming evidence that

an overactive or sluggish thyroid can greatly affect mood and metabolism.

While there is much debate among the medical community about the exact definition of over- or underactive thyroid, there is no debate that too much or too little of the thyroid hormones will cause either depression or anxiety in the patient. Most medical doctors also hold that anxiety or depression will not be the only signs of a thyroid disorder.

Goiters

A goiter is an enlargement of the thyroid gland on one or both sides of the neck. Remember, your thyroid gland is shaped like a butterfly with its body lying in front of the trachea and its wings spread out on either side of your throat. When this enlargement happens, you can easily see the goiter as a mass on your neck. Typically, these growths are malignant and not caused by over- or underproduction of the thyroid hormones.

Goiters may be caused by diet or a lack of iodine; however these are extremely rare causes due to the quality of most American diets today and the abundance of iodine in the typical diet. The most common cause of goiters can be blamed on the pituitary gland and the overproduction of Thyroid Stimulating Hormone (TSH).

This condition is more common in women than in men and may take years to fully manifest. Fortunately, many patients find that treating the pituitary gland and reducing the levels of TSH work well at reducing or eliminating the goiter. In rare cases, surgery may be the only option for patients depending on the size and location of the goiter especially if the goiter is pressing against the trachea or esophagus making breathing or eating difficult.

Hyperthyroidism

For some people, their thyroid gland over produces the hormones and chemicals needed for healthy body function. These patients suffer from hyperthyroidism, or overactive thyroid. Patients may experience sudden, unexplained weight loss or may experience a drastic increase in overall body metabolism. They may also experience rapid heartbeats, uncontrolled sweating, irritability, or nervousness. (All common symptoms of anxiety!!)

In addition to these symptoms, patients with hyperthyroidism may suffer from increased appetite, tremors in the hands and/or feet, sensitivity to heat, irritable bowel syndrome, changes in menstrual cycles, and thinning skin. Do not take these signs lightly. If left untreated, some patients have developed Grave's ophthalmopathy which may cause long term eye problems and impair vision.

There may be several causes for an overactive thyroid, You may have an inflamed thyroid which causes stored hormones to leak into the bloodstream unexpectedly. A common cause for hyperthyroidism is Grave's disease. Goiters, Plummer's disease, and toxic adenoma may also be contributing factors.

Most physicians will prescribe beta blockers or anti-thyroid medications to treat hyperthyroidism. These may be prescribed individually or in a combination. Patients usually see results within six weeks. Unfortunately, the anti-thyroid medication has been known to cause liver disease so if your doctor prescribes this type of medication, be very cautious and monitor liver functions regularly.

Hypothyroidism

Also known as underactive thyroid, patients with hypothyroidism suffer when the thyroid gland does not produce enough hormones to properly regulate body chemistry. This condition is most often present in women over the age of 60. Patients may be asymptomatic in the early stages of the condition but persistent signs will develop over time if left untreated. This is one of the causes of my anxiety although I am far from the age in which it usually shows up.

There are a number of risk factors which may contribute to hypothyroidism. Patients who have had surgery in or around the thyroid area may develop hypothyroidism as a result. Patients who have been treated for hyperthyroidism may develop the condition later in life. Medications and radiation treatments to the throat area have been known to cause the condition. Additionally, anyone diagnosed with Hashimoto's thyroiditis, an inflammatory autoimmune condition, will often be diagnosed with hypothyroidism. Some doctors estimate that as many as 90% of patients with hypothyroidism have Hashimoto's Disease even though the test results may appear normal.

While not as common, there are other causes for the disorder. Some patients are born with hypothyroidism. These patients will appear normal at birth but will suffer from defective or underdeveloped thyroid glands. As a result, most states now require newborn thyroid screenings to check for unseen thyroid issues. Some women develop the condition during pregnancy. Hypothyroidism may also be brought on due to a pituitary gland issue or iodine deficiency.

Patients with hypothyroidism may mistake some of the signs and symptoms with those of normal aging, but it is important to speak with your doctor if you have a combination of multiple signs. Symptoms include fatigue, pain and stiffness in joints, thinning hair, impaired memory, dry skin, heavier than normal menstrual cycles, constipation, unexplained weight gain, elevated cholesterol levels, muscle weakness, or hoarseness.

Standard medicine treats hypothyroidism with a prescription of a synthetic thyroid hormone levothyroxine. This form of treatment typically takes approximately two weeks to absorb into the body. However, some patients report side effects to this treatment including heart palpitations, insomnia, and increased appetite. An alternative to this treatment is a natural extract containing both thyroxine and triiodothyronine. These extracts are available by prescription only.

Parathyroid

While not considered a major member of the endocrine system, the parathyroid gland does play a substantial role in the body's regulation of mood and anxiety. Located in the neck just behind the thyroid, your parathyroid glands (you have 4!) control the calcium in your body. These glands are only the size of a grain of rice yet they are vitally important to your nervous and neurological systems.

When most people think about calcium, they instantly think about milk commercials and strong bones. That's an important part of what calcium does, but it isn't the only role it plays in your body. Calcium acts as the primary conductor of electricity for the nervous system. The nervous system uses electrical impulses to send messages throughout the body. Calcium allows this process to take place. Without an adequate amount of calcium, or if the calcium isn't properly absorbed, processed, and distributed throughout the body, your body will become sluggish, weak and easily tired. Additional signs of calcium deficiency may include muscle spasms, memory loss, depression, hallucinations, and tingling in the hands and feet.

Despite the name, parathyroid glands are not directly related to the thyroid. They act as separate entities whose only function is to regulate calcium in the body. They do this be producing and secreting a hormone known as Parathyroid Hormone (PTH).

Hyperparathyroidism

For the vast majority of patients, issues from the parathyroid come from an overproduction of PTH. This may be caused by several factors including parathyroid adenoma, tumors, or a malfunction of the parathyroid. In such cases, the body may have excess or too little calcium to properly function.

Patients may have hyperparathyroidism for years without symptoms severe enough to cause alarm. It has often been linked to osteoporosis and kidney stones. In more severe cases, patients may suffer from impaired memory, forgetfulness, depression, abdominal pain, joint pain, fatigue, loss of appetite, nausea, and overall body weakness.

Many patients, particularly older women, find that hormone replacement therapy works well in treating the symptoms of hyperparathyroidism, although this treatment has been shown to increase the risk of breast cancer so you will need to work closely with your doctor if you choose this type of therapy. Another common treatment is the prescription of biphosphonates to help with the absorption of calcium in the body. Some patients have reported fever, vomiting, and low blood pressure with this treatment.

Hypoparathyroidism

A less common, though far more serious condition, is hypoparathyroidism. This condition is very rare. With this condition, the body produces and secretes unusually low levels of PTH.

Symptoms for this condition often mimic other illnesses. Signs include headaches; depression; mood swings; tingling in the hands and feet; muscle spasms in the face, hands, legs, and feet; painful menstruation; memory loss; and fatigue. In some cases, patients have reported difficulty breathing and seizures.

If left untreated, hypoparathyroidism may cause several irreversible health conditions including stunted growth (particularly if the condition is present in children), impaired mental development, calcium deposits on the brain, and cataracts. Additionally, but reversible, conditions may also include grand mal seizures, impaired kidney functions, and heart arrhythmias.

Treatment for this condition often includes calcium supplements and increased vitamin D. Patients will often be placed on a strict diet to increase calcium levels while decreasing the amount of phosphorus in the body. Some doctors may prescribe PTH replacement therapy although, as of this writing, that treatment has not been approved by the FDA.

Pituitary Gland

No larger than a pea, the pituitary gland is a giant in your body's endocrine system. As mentioned before, it produces and secretes TSH. It is also responsible for adrenocorticotropic hormone (ACTH). That hormone controls the secretion of cortisol within the body and controls the body's fight or flight response.

The pituitary gland has been called the master gland because it controls the production and secretion of hormones by other glands in the body. It works closely with the hypothalamus. The hypothalamus sends signals to the pituitary gland to stimulate or reduce hormone production and pituitary glands responds accordingly. The pituitary gland also works very closely with the thyroid.

In addition to TSH and ACTH, the pituitary gland also produces Follicle Stimulating Hormone (FSH), Growth Hormone (GH), Luteinizing Hormone (LH), and Prolactin. These hormones are essential in maintaining the healthy and normal function of the testes and the ovaries as well as ensuring the healthy growth of the body through childhood and adolescence.

Hypopituitarism

Patients who have hypopituitarism suffer from the pituitary gland either not producing or under producing one or more major hormone. It is a progressive condition that often builds for years unrecognized until the symptoms become overwhelming. Then, patients feel what they believe to be a sudden onset of the condition.

Symptoms may include a number of signs that are easily confused with normal aging or with other less serious conditions. Patients may feel fatigue, reduced sexual desire, or sensitivity to the cold. They may experience decreased appetite and weight loss. They may also have facial puffiness, anemia, or suffer from infertility.

Anyone with a family history of hypopituitarism may be at risk for the condition. However, it is most often the result of injury, stroke, tumor growth on the pituitary gland, or infections.

The most common treatment for the disorder is hormonal replacement therapy which may be a lifelong option for many patients. It must be noted however, that this type of hormonal therapy can result in an imbalance of other hormones within the body. Some patients see an excessive production of cortisol while taking these therapies. If the condition is a result of a tumor or growth on the pituitary gland, your physician may recommend surgery or radiation depending on the severity of the case.

Did You Know?

The American Cancer Society estimates that 10,000 new cases of pituitaries tumors are diagnosed each year. Some 1 in 4 adults may be living with a pituitary tumor without realizing it.

Fortunately, the vast majority of these tumors are benign adenomas. Most patients remain asymptomatic for years and only discover the condition as part of testing for other conditions usually as part of an MRI scan.

Pancreas

Your pancreas is a gland roughly six inches in length that site behind the stomach in the abdominal cavity. It produces and secretes hormones directly responsible for digestion and blood glucose regulation. Without the pancreas, you would not be able to digest your food properly or would have difficulty regulating salt and gastric acids.

There are five major hormones that the pancreas is responsible for producing: gastrin, glucagon, insulin, somatostatin, and vasoactive intestinal peptide (VIP). These hormones work together to ensure that food is properly digested and nutrients are absorbed into the body. They work directly with the digestive system in all stages of food breakdown.

The pancreas produces and secretes insulin, the primary hormone responsible for the regulation of blood glucose within the body. The most common issue directly relating to insulin production and secretion is diabetes but some individuals suffer from pre-diabetic conditions such as hyperglycemia and hypoglycemia. We will be discussing these conditions in more detail in Chapter 8.

Pancreatitis

Pancreatitis is an inflammation of the pancreas that directly affects the production of pancreatic hormones. Cases of inflammation may be acute and severe requiring immediate medical attention or may be mild and go away without any medical treatment at all.

Symptoms will vary depending on the severity of the condition but may include any of the following symptoms either individually or in combination: abdominal pain in the upper region that radiates to the back, nausea, vomiting, an abdomen that's tender to the touch, pain that increases after eating, unexplained weight loss, or oily stools.

Pancreatitis occurs when digestive enzymes are released in the pancreas causing damage to the gland. These enzymes are normally only released inside the digestive tract which has an interior lining strong enough to handle their acidic nature. The pancreas is not designed to handle such acidity. Several conditions may cause this premature secretion such as alcoholism, family history, hyperparathyroidism, gallstones, smoking, and cystic fibrosis.

Pancreatitis can cause some serious complications if left untreated for too long. It can cause pockets, known as pseudocysts, to form inside the pancreas. Infections and breathing difficulties may occur. Patients may develop diabetes or kidney failure as the result of this condition. Lastly, patients may suffer from bouts of malnutrition or develop pancreatic cancer.

As you can see pancreatitis is a serious condition not to be trifled with. The treatment usually requires admittance into a hospital for careful monitoring. While in the medical facility, patients will fast for several days to allow the pancreas to recover from the symptoms. Intravenous fluids and electrolytes will be given to ensure the patient does not become dehydrated. Additionally, medication to treat the condition will be given through the IV.

Testes

The testes, or testicles as they are more commonly referred to, are located directly behind the penis in all males. They're small (only about the size of a large grape) and held within the scrotum. Due to their location, they are fairly exposed to potential damage through injury but this positioning in the body allows them to remain at cooler temperatures than other organs and glands. Lower temperatures are fundamental for healthy sperm development.

The testes are responsible for the development of sperm and testosterone. They control how the secretion of testosterone into the body. In order to effectively know how much testosterone the body needs, the testes rely on input from hypothalamus and pituitary glands. Those glands send hormones to the testicles to stimulate or reduce testosterone production. They are the primary reproductive organ in all men. Without these glands, men would not develop the typical male traits such as muscle mass, body and facial hair, and a deeper voice.

The testicles most often malfunction due to injury or a physical abnormality at birth. While many physical problems dealing with the testicles can be corrected through non-invasive surgical procedures, there may still be a chance that infertility may arise depending on the severity of the individual case. A man suffering from this issue may also require testosterone hormone therapy as we'll discuss a little later in the chapter.

Ovaries

Just as the testes are vital to the male reproductive system, so too are the ovaries equally, if not more, important to the female anatomy. The ovaries produce and control the secretion of two vital hormones – estrogen and progesterone. They also produce egg development in women. Like their male counterpart, these hormones are responsible for the development of the female body including breast development, menstruation, and conception.

The ovaries are about the same size as the testicles but are located inside the abdominal cavity on either side of the uterus. Fallopian tubes connect the ovaries to the uterus. During a woman's monthly cycle, the ovaries will release the eggs through the fallopian tubes into the uterus where they will either be fertilized by the sperm or will be discarded out of the body. In order to accomplish this task, the ovaries regulate the secretion of estrogen and progesterone throughout the cycle to ensure maximum fertility.

Unfortunately, there are a number of conditions and illnesses that can interfere with this sensitive process. Endometriosis, fibroids, cysts, cancer, diabetes, and high blood pressure can all wreak havoc on the normal activities of the ovaries. We will be discussing some of these conditions further in Chapter 8, but for now we will concentrate primarily on the condition which most affects anxiety and mood.

Polycystic Ovarian Syndrome

Research suggests that there is a direct link between Polycystic Ovarian Syndrome (PCOS) and the elevated rate of anxiety in women. As the name implies, women who suffer from this condition have numerous cysts in and around their ovaries. These cysts may be tiny and cause few side effects or may be substantial in size and cause infertility, emotional imbalance, and abdominal pain. In the vast majority of cases, women are asymptomatic for years and only discover the problem as a result of infertility.

Most doctors believe that PCOS causes a disruption in the production and secretion of estrogen and progesterone. The ovaries may be receiving the required data from the hypothalamus and pituitary glands; however, the ovaries are unable to respond accordingly. As a result, the over or under produce the necessary hormones.

Women who suffer from this condition may have any number of symptoms that go unrecognized for years. Signs may include irregular monthly cycles, weight gain, unusual hair growth, or severe acne.

Treatment for this condition usually requires surgical removal. Fortunately, new advances in medicine allow for this procedure to be completed by less invasive techniques. Most physicians will use a procedure called laparoscopy to remove the cysts from the ovaries. Patients suffer little down time with this procedure and are back home within a few hours after surgery. They may resume normal routines within a few days of the surgery.

Hypothalamus

Many scientists and physicians believe the hypothalamus is the most essential gland in the entire endocrine system. It acts as the regulator, controlling the overall balance, or homeostasis, within the body. It also acts as the direct link between the endocrine and nervous systems.

It's located in the brain between the pituitary gland and the thalamus gland and is roughly the size of an almond. And it packs quite a punch for such a little package! Your heart rate, blood pressure, appetite, body weight, electrolyte balances, sleep cycles, and body temperature are all directly related to the function of the hypothalamus gland. Additionally, it works directly with the pituitary gland to regulate the production and secretion of pituitary hormones.

It is this close working relationship and close proximity to the pituitary gland which often causes difficulties for doctors when determining the underlying cause for a glandular or hormonal problem. Fortunately, by modifying the hormonal tests to specifically target hormones produced in the hypothalamus, doctors can often rule out the pituitary gland and narrow down the condition at hand.

Hypothalamic Disease

The most common case of this disorder is some type of physical injury to the brain which directly affects the hypothalamus and its hormone production although other diseases and circulatory problems may also cause the disorder. Patients with hypothalamic disease often experience problems with appetite or sleep disorders. Additionally, patients may experience issues with hormones produced in the pituitary gland due to the close relationship of the two glands.

Patients may experience increased weight gain or may be overweight and have difficulty losing weight regardless of diet or exercise. They may suffer from abnormal body temperature, sleep difficulty, impaired vision, loss of hair, or dizziness. Fatigue and increased urination have also been reported. Lastly, hypothalamic disease has been known to cause or be associated with hypothyroidism.

Depending on the cause of the condition, hormone replace therapy may be a viable option for patients. This is a particularly helpful treatment option for problems within the hypothalamus not caused by scarring, injury, or tumors. If a physical malformation is the cause, your doctor may suggest surgery to correct the issue.

Pineal Gland

Shaped like a pine cone and only a third of an inch big, the pineal gland has long been a mystery to the endocrine system. The French philosopher, Rene Descartes, once referred to is at the brain's third eye believing it was the primary location of the soul. That explanation has now been ruled out by modern science.

The pineal gland is responsible for the body's production of melatonin and plays a major function in the body's natural sleep rhythm. We will discuss the importance of melatonin momentarily. The pineal gland is not known to produce any other hormones.

Adrenal Glands

These small, triangular glands are located on top of the kidneys and produce the hormones epinephrine, norepinephrine, cortisone, cortisol, and aldostrone. These hormones are responsible for the body's metabolism, reaction to stress, and blood pressure. They are also responsible for the production of sex hormones in both men and women.

There are two adrenal glands in the human body, each located on top of a kidney. These glands are tiny, measuring only one and a half by three inches. Despite their tiny size they control and secrete numerous hormones essential for normal life. When it fails to function properly, these activities may be negatively impacted.

Adrenal Fatigue

Adrenal fatigue is a syndrome in which the adrenal glands function at a much lower rate than required by your body. This condition can make it difficult for suffers to get out of bed each day and virtually impossible to function properly.

Symptoms of the condition include a general tiredness or blah feeling. Many suffers are highly susceptible to infections and illnesses. They may have frequent colds or the flu several times throughout the year. Many of the signs mimic depression. Most patients report needing a stimulant, usually coffee, cola, or some other form of caffeine just to get the day started.

Stress is known to increase the likelihood of adrenal fatigue. Patients who suffer prolonged stress or crisis situations are at a greater risk for the condition. Poor diet, lack of exercise, and loss of sleep also contribute to the condition.

Adrenal Failure (Addison's Disease)

Also known as adrenal insufficiency, adrenal failure is more complex than adrenal fatigue. Adrenal failure can be divided up into two distinct categories, primary adrenal failure and secondary adrenal failure. With primary adrenal failure, or Addison's Disease, the adrenal glands are physically damaged and cannot produce enough cortisol for the body. In secondary adrenal failure, the problem occurs when the pituitary gland fails to produce enough ACTH to stimulate cortisol production in the adrenal glands.

The most common signs of adrenal failure are chronic fatigue, unexplained weight loss, loss of appetite, muscle weakness, and abdominal pain. Other symptoms may include sudden drop in blood pressure, nausea, vomiting, diarrhea, hypoglycemia, headaches, uncontrolled sweating, loss of sexual desire, craving of salty foods, and irregular menstrual cycles.

If left untreated, adrenal failure could worsen and develop into adrenal crisis which is life threatening. If you have any of the symptoms listed here that suddenly worsen without explanation, contact medical help immediately.

Know Your Hormones

There are over four dozen hormones found in the human body. Each one is regulating different functions. Remember our chat room scenario above. You can imagine how confusing the conversation can be with each one chatting about a different function at the same time.

While each hormone is important to the regulation of proper body functions, for the purposes of our discussion we will be focusing on the hormones which deal most directly with mood and anxiety. Some we have already mentioned but they deserve special attention to fully understand their importance when dealing with anxiety issues. For additional information on other hormones not covered here, you may want to visit the U.S. National Library of Medicine by the National Institutes of Health (www.nlm.nih.gov/medlineplus/hormones.html).

Estrogen

One of the most well-known and widely discussed of all hormones, estrogen is actually a group of several hormones that have a profound effect on a woman's body. This hormone group is primarily made up of estrone, estradiol, and estriol but does include several other minor hormones as well. While both men and women have estrogenic hormones in their bodies, it is unclear how great a role these hormones play in men.

Estrogen is responsible for the development of female sexual characteristics in women. Produced in the ovaries, adrenal glands, and within fat tissues, these hormones control breast and uterine development, a woman's monthly menstrual cycle, conception and pregnancy, and fetal development. In addition, estrogen helps regulate heart and liver function, bone density, brain development and function, and metabolic processes within women.

Women who suffer from low estrogen or experience premenopausal symptoms may suffer from infertility issues, delayed puberty in teens, irregular menstrual cycles, mood swings, anxiety, and depression. For many women, hormone replace therapy is a good alternative particularly in dealing with infertility issues however; prolonged estrogen replacement therapy has been linked to increase risks of stroke, heart attack, and breast cancer.

Progesterone

Like estrogen, progesterone plays a major role in regulating the menstrual cycles of women. This hormone also helps ready a woman's body for pregnancy. Women who have progesterone deficiencies may find it difficult or impossible to conceive without some type of fertility treatment.

Produced in the ovaries, the adrenal gland, and in the placenta of pregnant women, progesterone is to stimulate the secretion of proteins during her monthly cycle to prepare her body for conception. If conception does not take place, the progesterone levels, along with the estrogen levels will drop completing the menstruation portion of the cycle.

Women who suffer from low progesterone levels may notice symptoms including irritability, moodiness, headaches, depression, fatigue, low sex drive, difficulty focusing on tasks, memory impairment, weight gain, infertility, miscarriages, and vaginal irritation.

Several treatment options exist for these patients. Oral progesterone supplements may be prescribed particularly in causes of fertility treatments or in preparation of in vitro fertilization. Some women find that topical progesterone gels and creams are very effective at increasing hormonal levels. It's interesting to note that progesterone is often used to ease the withdrawal symptoms of patients who are discontinuing the use of certain drugs such as benzodiazepines.

Testosterone

Testosterone is the hormone responsible for men becoming men. While both men and women have testosterone in the body, it is the hormone that determines whether a child will become male in the womb. Produced in the testes, it is directly responsible for sperm production and sex drive in men as well as predominantly male characteristics such as body and facial hair and muscle development.

Testosterone levels in men generally begin to fall after the age of 40 with most men experiencing a 1.6% drop in levels annually. For men whose levels drop at a more drastic rate, they may have a condition known as hypogonadism in which the testosterone level drops to levels more common in men 20 years or more their senior. In such cases, men may experience severe symptoms that affect mood and cognitive function.

There may be several reasons for a lower level of testosterone in man at an early age. There may be an issue with the testes or there may be a malfunction of the pituitary gland and the release of a luteinizing hormone (LH) which regulates the level of testosterone in the body.

Symptoms of low testosterone levels include loss of hair, depression, moodiness, fatigue, anger, decreased muscle mass, loss of sexual desire, reduced cognitive powers, and an increase in abdominal fat. Unfortunately, many men who experience these symptoms often attribute them as a normal part of aging.

Melatonin

Most of us are well familiar with that relaxed, drowsy feeling after a large Thanksgiving dinner. That's because turkey is full of the natural chemical melatonin, a hormone that helps regulate sleep cycles. Humans produce melatonin in the pineal gland.

Your body has a unique internal clock that determines when you sleep and when you wake. For most people, melatonin levels are highest in the evening and nighttime hours and lowest during the day. This cycle will be reversed for those who work at night and sleep during the day. Light will increase the production of melatonin which helps explain why the largest levels can be found at the end of the day. This reliance on light may also help explain why some people develop a winter depression during the winter months when the days are shorter.

Melatonin supplements are beneficial for most people who suffer from insomnia as a safe alternative to a prescription sleep aid. That being said, women who are pregnant or nursing and children should not take these supplements without first consulting with a physician. Fortunately, melatonin supplements can be for both long- and short-term durations without adverse effects.

Cortisol

You've probably seen the commercials on TV promising a miracle diet cure that lowers your body cortisol levels and instantly sheds unwanted pounds. You may have even been tempted, in a middle of a sleepless night, to try this wonder pill. But cortisol is more than just a hormone that can cause weight gain. It is the master stress hormone!

Cortisol belongs to glucocorticoids class of hormones. These types of hormones affect almost every other organ in the human body. Scientists know that it regulate insulin use; controls the body's response to stress; helps create a sense of emotional balance and well-being; regulates blood pressure; and helps control metabolism. That being said, they believe it may control or influence many more functions that they are not currently aware of.

Like some other hormones in the body, cortisol levels fluctuate throughout the day depending on the numerous factors. Ideally, the levels should follow a natural rhythm with the lowest levels found at night during your sleep, spiking in the morning as you begin the day and need an added boost of energy, and gradually tapering off during the day with occasional mini increases seen as stress levels rise. By the end of the day, your cortisol levels should be back to the lower end of the spectrum to allow your body to rest.

Unfortunately, most people live under a constant amount of stress that the body must process and control. Increased stress leads to increased cortisol levels which lead to a plethora of health conditions such as obesity, high blood pressure, diabetes, anxiety disorder, depression, Alzheimer's disease, and chronic fatigue.

However, stress may not be the only reason for elevated cortisol levels. High levels of cortisol may indicate a problem with the adrenal glands or with pituitary glands which release ACTH. A malfunction in either gland can cause cortisol levels to spike.

Symptoms for those who have elevated cortisol levels include headaches, ulcers, unexplained weight gain, reduced sexual interest, moodiness, depression, anxiety, food cravings, irregular menstrual cycles, insomnia, and increased body fat.

Balance in All Things

As you can see, hormones and the endocrine system play a major role in all the functions of the body especially in determining mood, depression, and anxiety. These hormones must work together in perfect harmony; otherwise your body will be out of balance and you will experience a wide range of physical and emotional symptoms.

Hormonal imbalances may be caused by external factors such as stress or may be caused by a problem with the endocrine system itself. Made up of eight glands, these glands use an internal feedback system to self regulate the production of almost 50 different hormones used by the body on a daily basis. If one cog in the system is broken or impaired, the entire system will suffer.

My Hormonal Hell!

I've had a long history of hormonal issues that I attributed to hormonal changes during my monthly cycle. Each month about ten days before my period would began I would be plagued with terrible anxiety and sometimes even panic attacks.

In 2012 at the age of 36, while trying to taper off Xanax, I sought the medical guidance of a new general doctor. He in turn suggested I have a complete hormonal analysis, which I did and the test results showed that my progesterone, testosterone, and DHEA levels were all on the low side of the normal and nowhere near optimal ranges, especially for someone my age. He elaborated on what optimal levels were and also expressed that my thyroid results were on the low as well. It was recommended that I begin hormone replacement therapy. To say I was reluctant was an understatement. Here I was desperately trying to come off one medicine and now this doctor wanted to start me on several new medications. After going and getting a second opinion, it was confirmed that my levels were indeed off and hormone replacement therapy was the best option for me.

From past experiences I learned rather quickly that you should only start one new thing at a time. So the first hormone I started taking was oral bio-identical progesterone. I was reluctant because of the research I had done on the use of progesterone suggested its effects and withdrawals were similar to that of a benzo. I mean here I was desperately fighting to come off the hardest drug known to man to taper, A BENZO, to then turn around and replace it with a similar medication.

I was really nervous to say the least, but the more I researched the more I realized that yes they are similar, but they both affect the GABA receptor sites in a different way. Which I'm not going to get into now. So I followed my doctor's advice and began the treatment.

In the beginning of the treatment I was sleeping better, however I was experiencing more anxiety during the day and when I expressed my concerns to my general doctor he couldn't understand how the two could correlate with one another. So I took my business elsewhere and found a wonderful doctor that practices integrative and functional medicine, with a specialty in bioidentical hormones.

I'm so glad I did because she ran other tests on me and found out I had HIGH cortisol and that is why I was experiencing more anxiety from the progesterone. You see, cortisol suppresses progesterone production and secretion, but high progesterone levels can increase cortisol production and secretion. Yes, my progesterone levels were low, but part of the cause was due to high cortisol levels. I was actually making the condition worse by increasing the progesterone in my system and producing MORE cortisol.

I stumbled upon this great piece that I'd like to share with all of you:

> "Initially, most women feel a calming effect when they use progesterone. However, after approximately eight months of high active progesterone levels a clinical depression may develop. Often times the cause of this depression is not attributed to the use of the progesterone cream. The second downside of high active progesterone is its effect on active cortisol levels in the body . . . High levels of active progesterone . . . cause a significant increase in free active cortisol . . . High active cortisol over the long term can result in hunger and sugar or carbohydrate cravings, weight gain around the waist, reduced muscle mass, bone thinning, food sensitivities and allergies, reduced athletic endurance, yeast overgrowth, reduced thyroid function, insomnia, PMS, and if not corrected, eventual exhaustion and chronic fatigue." (Gabriel)

My new doctor worked with me to lower my

cortisol levels with supplements and by lowering the progesterone I was taking. From this, my cortisol levels came down and I felt much better. Let me be perfectly clear, the progesterone I was taking did not cause me to have high cortisol. I already had high cortisol from the lifestyle choice I made (my job, my gym training, etc). What progesterone did was to aggravate the situation because it didn't accurately address the root cause of my hormonal imbalance. Hormonal harmony is a tricky subject to master. It may take some time to find the right combination and treatment options for you. But be persistent and thorough in your quest and you can feel better!

Gabriel, E. (n.d.). *THE PROBLEM OF EXCESS PROGESTERONE*. Retrieved from The Green Willow Tree: http://www.greenwillowtree.com/Page.bok?file=wildyam.html

Chapter 3 Understanding Neurotransmitters

As we learned in Chapter 2, hormones control the chemical functions of many of the body's activities. Neurotransmitters work in a similar fashion. They are the chemical messengers of the body sent out by the brain to ensure the body is functioning properly.

There are two types of neurotransmitters in the body, excitatory and inhibitory. Excitatory neurotransmitters are excited to be on their journey because they are there to produce an action of some kind. Inhibitory neurotransmitters are just the opposite. They are attempted to stop an action of some sort. Each type of neurotransmitter will only work with a like receptor. For example, an inhibitory neurotransmitter will not communicate with an excitatory receptor. The lock must fit the key.

If at any time there is a depletion of neurotransmitters in the body or if there is a problem with the communication between neurotransmitters, bodily functions can be greatly impaired. Nutrition, diet, substance abuse, stress and pollution have all been known to diminish the levels of neurotransmitters in the body. What's more, certain types of medications, such as those regularly prescribed for anxiety interfere with the functions of the neurotransmitters in our bodies. It was a painful discovery when I learned that my GABA neurotransmitters had been damaged due to my longstanding prescription of Xanax. The medicine doctors said would help with anxiety was preventing my body from controlling the anxiety naturally.

Neurotransmitters and Anxiety

It turns out your brain is the source of your anxiety, both physically and emotionally. Just as the negative and anxiety thoughts begin in the mind, so too do the physical reactions and symptoms that accompany those thoughts. The neurotransmitters in your brain send out electric impulses that signal the response of the organs and glands in your body. These impulses can increase production of hormones such as cortisol or decrease production of melatonin making it difficult to sleep. Your brain and the responses in it, ultimately determine heart rate, blood pressure, and breathing. To understand how that is possible, we must fully understand the roles key neurotransmitters play.

Epinephrine (Adrenaline)

Epinephrine, also known as adrenaline, is the well as known fight or flight neurotransmitter. It controls who the body deals with an immediate threat. When adrenaline is released in the body, your brain instantly knows there is danger about and responds with fear, including increased heart rate, difficulty breathing, and sweating. These are all the same symptoms of an anxiety attack.

It's an effective system designed to save us from life threatening situations. Image if you were in the building on fire. Your adrenaline would ramp up production and encourage you to find an exit quickly.

Unfortunately, your body can't tell the difference between an emotional threat and a physical one. Furthermore the symptoms of an anxiety attack and the release of adrenaline are almost identical. When we suffer an anxiety attack, the body releases more adrenaline which increases our fear and anxiety. It's a somewhat vicious circle.

Norepineprhine

Norepinephrine has two major roles. First, it relays messages to the brain in the body's fight or flight response. Second, it prepares the brain for environmental stimulants. Without norepinephrine, your body would never feel pain or emotions. Imagine you're walking alone to your car one evening and hear a noise. Your senses immediately perk up to determine whether the noise is friend or foe. That's the norepinephrine in your body activating to alert your brain to a potentially dangerous situation. It's instanteous.

Interestingly, the release of norepinephrine in the brain seems to alter with experience. As we learn and recognize different dangers, the triggers modify so that or bodies naturally eliminate most 'safe' situations. That is what keeps us from feeling that instant alertness that leads to anxiety and panic.

Unfortunately, when the amount of norepinephrine is low, our bodies compensate by releasing more adrenaline in the system. It acts as a protective mechanism to prevent harm. It also induces anxiety because the levels of norepinephrine are not adequate to counteract the stimuli in our system.

Dopamine

Dopamine is a major neurotransmitter which helps the areas of the brain communicate with one another. This chemical is responsible for the moods you normally feel. It creates the feel good, happy moods as well as the anxious, depressed, and irritable moods. It works directly in the decision making process and affects how the brain processes information to form a plan of action.

When dopamine levels are balanced and in harmony with the rest of our body we feel calm and at peace with the world. We may be happy and content with our lives. Usually there's an even keel to our emotional status during that time. When levels are elevated, we feel a sense of euphoria and uncontrolled happiness. Unfortunately, when levels are low, we tend to feel depressed and anxious regardless of the situation.

Researchers believe that dopamine levels are directly related to diet and nutrition. While no actual foods contain dopamine, our diets can directly influence to body's production of dopamine. As we'll see in Chapter 5, the right foods can make all the difference in the world in dopamine production.

> **Did You Know?**
>
> A one hour massage has been shown to increase the levels of both serotonin and dopamine. Research shows serotonin levels will increase by an average of 28% and dopamine by some 31%. Another great reason to treat yourself to a spa day.

Endorphins

Endorphins are the neurotransmitters responsible for pain suppression, euphoria, appetite, and sexual desire. There are approximately 20 different types of endorphins residing in the pituitary gland.

If you've ever spent time in a gym, you've heard the term endorphins thrown around regularly. They are what's responsible for what many people call a 'runner's high.' Athletes often report a feeling of euphoria after a particularly strenuous exercise routine. Scientists do not fully understand the complexities of endorphin release, but there is little doubt that they play a major role in athletic success.

As with all things in the body, the release of endorphins is highly individualized. Two people can experience the exact same physical stimulus and experience drastically different levels of pain.

There are several ways to increase the release of endorphins even without a trip to the gym. Massage therapy has been shown to increase endorphins. Meditation can trigger their release as well. Lastly, sex has been proven to release as many endorphins as a good workout.

Serotonin

Serotonin is created in the brain from the conversion of several building proteins. Although it does all its work in the brain, it is stored in the digestive tract and in blood platelets throughout the body.

Serotonin acts as the primary neurotransmitter in the brain. It sends out electronic signals from one region of the brain to another allowing those regions to communicate directly with each other. It is estimated that every brain cell, all 40 million of them, are affected by serotonin in some manner. It plays a major role in body functions such as our cardiovascular system, muscular development, and the endocrine system. Additionally, brain cells that are responsible for mood, sleep regulation, appetite, memory and sexual desire all utilize serotonin throughout the course of the day.

Serotonin has long been thought to be a vital player in depression and anxiety. While researchers have yet to discover the exact connection between the chemical and the psychological conditions, it is believed that low serotonin levels or an interruption in the communication from one area of the brain to the other cause radical mood swings such as OCD, anger, panic, anxiety, and depression.

As of yet, there are no effective ways to actually measure serotonin levels in a living brain. It is possible to measure the levels in the blood, but we have no way of knowing if that amount is actually in the brain being utilized or is merely being stored for future use. Because of this, scientists still have many unanswered questions about the internal processes serotonin performs in the brain.

Another question scientists are pondering is determining the order of events in relation to serotonin levels and mood shifts. Does the drop in serotonin levels cause anxiety and depression or do the serotonin levels drop because of anxiety and depression? The answer to that question could hold major implications in the world of anxiety treatment.

Diet plays a role in the production of serotonin levels in the body. There is no known food that contains serotonin, but there are foods that encourage the production of serotonin in the body. We'll discuss those more in Chapter 5. Likewise, there are substances that interrupt the production of serotonin causing massive side effects. We'll cover those in more detail in Chapter 6.

While men and women both have serotonin, men generally have a slightly higher amount than women. It is unclear exactly how female hormones such as estrogen and progesterone interact with serotonin but many researchers believe that this interaction may result in a greater number of anxiety problems for women.

Additionally, there is some research that suggests there may be a link between neurotransmitters such as serotonin and dementia and Alzheimer's disease. Scientists believe that the slowing of neurotransmitters is a natural part of the aging process which is accelerated in dementia patients. Definitive is still a long way off in that area.

Did You Know?

Although serotonin is produced in the brain and intestines, 80-90% of all serotonin in the body can be found in the intestinal tract.

GABA

Gamma-Amino Butyric Acid (GABA) is an inhibitor neurotransmitter that works to calm the effects of excess adrenaline and norepinephrine during times of stress and anxiety. Easily the most abundant inhibitor in the body, GABA is also responsible for inducing sleep, relaxing the body, and controlling motor functions. GABA has been used to treat epilepsy patients and has been successful in reducing tremors.

Low levels of GABA have been known to cause anxiety and stress in patients as there is nothing to counteract the effects of adrenaline and norepinephrine coursing through the body. Another common symptom of reduced levels is bouts of chronic pain.

While more information is needed on effectiveness of GABA supplements, many people currently use these supplements to relieve anxiety and tension, alleviate the symptoms of premenstrual syndrome (PMS), treat ADHD, relieve pain, and lower blood pressure. It is important to note that these supplements have not been thoroughly studied and no concrete evidence exists that proves these supplements have any effect at all on these conditions. Furthermore, there are no regulatory standards in place to ensure the quality of these supplements.

Calming Your Internal Family

As you can see, the central nervous system with all its many neurotransmitters works closely with the endocrine system we covered in Chapter 2. These two are the internal siblings charged with keeping your emotional life balance. When they work together in harmony, all is right with the world. When they disagree, you suffer anxiety, depression, sleeplessness, and drastic mood swings.

Remember, one system is not more important than the other. By understanding how the systems work together, you can make changes to your lifestyle and work closely with your physicians to ensure that both systems are balanced.

A Fight from Within

As I discussed in the last chapter, my doctor's had prescribed progesterone to correct hormonal issues I was experiencing but that treatment was hindered by my long term benzo use. I soon discovered that benzos directly affect the GABA function. Remember GABA acts as the inhibitor neurotransmitter. It's your internal tranquilizer. When you take benzos, as I had for many years, that function is taken over by the medication. The result was my GABA were shot. I was suffering from a decreased GABA inhibition and an increased excitability of the glutamate system. Needless to say, my central nervous system was completely out of whack!

Progesterone binds with GABA receptors in the central nervous system. These receptors are responsible for maintaining an appropriate mood. GABA receptors are the receptors to which antidepressant drugs and anti- anxiety drugs bind to produce their effects. Studies show that these mood-altering drugs work because they elevate the concentration of a progesterone by-product. Therefore, progesterone can be prescribed as a natural antidepressant and anti-anxiety treatment.

The benzos I was tapering off of and the progesterone I was taking an increased dose of were having a major disagreement right in the middle of my central nervous system and the fight revolved around GABA! I was not an enjoyable experience.

Chapter 4 Toxins in Our Mists

It may seem strange to think that we are exposed on a daily basis to toxins that kill and alter our moods, cause bouts of depression and anxiety, modify our brain chemistry, and influence breathing, heart rate, and other bodily functions. Yet that is exactly what is happening. In some cases (as we'll discuss shortly), the toxins are closer than you think. Right inside our own bodies. We are literally being poisoned from the inside as well as the outside.

I was horrified to learn about the dangers of amalgam fillings, which are still being used today despite repeated data that shows the negative effects they can have on patients. Only recently did the FDA issue warnings regarding these fillings and then the warnings were only for pregnant women and young children. What about the rest of us? I discovered that my body was being poisoned every day and that was contributing to the anxiety I felt. When coupled with the other toxins we routinely encounter, we can begin to see how real these dangers are and how much they can affect our everyday lives.

In this chapter, we'll take a look at some of those toxins and discuss the most effective methods for cleansing your life of these harmful substances. We'll take a look at exactly what kind of toll they are taking on our bodies and how they affect our mood and mental capacities. Lastly, we'll uncover the signs and symptoms of exposure so that you know what to look for.

Benzene

If you've ever sat in a traffic jam or been stuck in a drive thru line, then you have been exposed to benzene. Benzene is found in gasoline and crude oil, but is also a major component in many manufactured items such as plastics, dyes, detergents, and pesticides.

Benzene is a carcinogen and has been linked to leukemia and blood cancers. However, any type of prolonged exposure to this chemical can cause noticeable symptoms. You may begin to feel drowsy or fuzzy headed. You may experience breathing difficulty and throat irritation. These breathing problems may you're your body to produce protective hormones causing an anxiety episode. Prolonged, extreme exposure can cause seizures.

To avoid benzene exposure, skip the drive through and try to limit exposure through congested traffic. Consider telecommuting, if that is an option, or alternating your work schedule to travel during off peak hours. If you run outdoors in urban areas, you may need to alter your exercise schedule to ensure you are not inadvertently exposing your body to harmful chemicals in the pursuit of health.

Did You Know?

One of the simplest ways to reduce the levels of benzene in your life is by replacing all your plastic containers and bottles with glass!

BPA

Biphenol-A (SBA) is a chemical used in the manufacturing process of plastics. In use since the late 1950s, today manufacturers use over 3.6 million tons of BPA annually. It is also commonly used as a protective barrier in metal containers such as food cans. As you can imagine, that puts BPA pretty much everywhere our food happens to be.

Unfortunately, BPA is a highly toxic chemical created from synthetic estrogen. It is known to inhibit the endocrine system, impair brain function and neurotransmitters, and modify behavior.

So why in the world are we still using in with our food supply?

That's a good question. According to the Federal Drug Administration (FDA), the risk of BPA seeping into the food supply is minimal. They also believe that low levels of BPA are not harmful to the general population.

That being said, there is a growing movement which encourages BPA free living and detoxification. And the good news is that detoxification works. Studies have shown that individuals who eliminate canned and processed foods packaged in BPA free containers and switch to a fresh fruit and vegetable diet see a marked reduction in their BPA levels within a week. More research needs to be conducted in this area, but this would indicate you can take positive steps in vastly improving your health with just some simply dietary changes. (We'll discuss this more in Chapter 5.)

But be careful. BPA is lurking in some fairly hidden spots. In addition to plastics and food cans, you can find BPA in baby jars, commercial and grocery receipts, toilet paper, dental sealants, and in alcohol products such as beer and wine. To completely eliminate BPA from your life be mindful of the hidden BPA traps and make efforts to avoid those traps if at all possible.

Formaldehyde Poisoning

When many people think of formaldehyde they think of mortuaries and embalming fluid. While that is one use for formaldehyde, you may be surprised to learn that is also commonly used in the manufacturing of many building materials found in your home. In fact, there is a high probability that your home is exposing you to formaldehyde at this moment.

Some of the primary sources of formaldehyde in your home include paint, wallpaper, and carpets. Pressed wood, plywood, and particle boards are another major source. As these products are used more extensively in modular homes, the risk of formaldehyde exposure is significantly greater in mobile homes than in traditional foundation homes. Other sources may include permanent press clothing, tobacco smoke, smoke from fireplaces and wood burning stoves, and cosmetics like nail polishes and hair care products.

Formaldehyde is a known carcinogen. It has been linked to cancers of the nasal cavity, stomach, and leukemia. There is debate about whether the exposure levels commonly found in homes can directly contribute to the risk of cancer. Even if we don't count the risk of cancer, formaldehyde exposure can be very dangerous. It can cause breathing difficulties and lung irritations. Additional symptoms include nausea, skin irritations, allergic reactions, and chest tightness.

Ridding your home of formaldehyde is difficult but there are steps you can take to limit the risk of exposure. Designate your home as smoke free and clean out chimneys annually. Never idle your vehicle near your home. (This will also help prevent exposure to Benzene!) Stick with solid wood furniture instead of prefabricated pieces. They last longer and have much less risk of formaldehyde exposure. Allow new furniture to air out before it enters the home. Allow your home to ventilate regularly by opening the windows and letting fresh air into the home. Always ventilate the home during and immediately after painting projects. Lastly, buy only Low- or Zero-VOC paints. They meet the same standards as other commercially available paints without the excess toxins.

Mercury & Heavy Metal

Mercury is a completely natural element. It's found in a number of sources including the air we breathe, the water covering the earth, and the soil our plants go in. It is also found in fish and in shellfish. Animals that eat a high fish diet may also contain large amounts of mercury. There are three primary types of mercury which we will be discussing here. All can be dangerous but there differ in subtle ways.

For many people, any mercury they ingest comes primarily from fish or shellfish. High levels of mercury in the body can damage the lungs, heart, kidneys, immune system, and the brain. If mercury finds its way into the bodies of small children or unborn babies, it can permanently damage the nervous system. However, the effects of exposure will vary greatly depending on a number of factors including the age, physical condition, and health issues of the person who consumed the mercury; the type of mercury exposure; the duration of the exposure; and the method of exposure.

Methylmercury

Methylmercury is the type of mercury commonly found in fish and shellfish. This is not the liquid form of mercury that many people are familiar with but rather an element fish and shellfish acquire from their environment. Usually, the amount is strictly dependent on the type of fish, the environment, and the size of the fish however; there have been some instances in which outbreaks have occurred that jeopardized the health of large portions of the population, both adults and children alike.

Symptoms of methylmercury poisoning include damage to the nervous system and brain, difficulty with cognitive reasoning skills, memory impairment, difficult speaking and with language recognition, and an inability to focus on tasks at hand. In addition to these types of symptoms, those exposed may also experience changes in vision particularly with regard to peripheral vision, lack of muscle coordination and impairment, and tingling feelings in the hands, feet, or legs.

Elemental Mercury

This is the type of mercury most people are familiar with. It is mercury in its basic elemental form, a liquid silvery substance that some people refer to as 'quick silver.' Many people believe that mercury poisoning occurs through direct touch of the element but that is not the primary method of exposure. Elemental mercury usually enters the body through inhalation after a spill or leak.

Mercury, when exposed to the air, usually vaporizes slowly. It's a process that actually happens every day in nature with no adverse effects because the concentration of vapors in the air is extremely low. Mercury concentrations in the atmosphere are diluted in the mixture of other elements and chemicals in the air.

When exposed in a warm, confined environment, that vaporization process happens much more quickly. As a result, dangerous toxins are released into the air in concentrated amounts. Once these toxins are inhaled they attach to various cells in the body causing major debilitating side effects. Think about the amount of air in your kitchen and the level of heat generated while cooking dinner. If a mercury skill occurred there, the vaporization would happen far more quickly than it would outside and the vaporized particles would have far less space in which to dilute.

Signs of mercury exposure include unexplainable mood swings such as extreme shyness, irritability, and nervousness; headaches; tingling in the hands and feet; difficulty with mental cognitive tasks. These symptoms can occur even in cases of small exposure. People who have suffered extreme exposure to mercury may experience kidney or respiratory failure and even death.

Mercury Compounds

As the name implies, mercury compounds are alloys made with some concentration of mercury. They may be either organic (the kind found in fish) or inorganic (elemental). Both organic and inorganic mercury compounds can be harmful if consumed or ingested.

Both forms of mercury compound enter the body through the gastrointestinal tract, yet organic are absorbed into the body more quickly than inorganic compounds. Symptoms of exposure may include memory loss, skin irritations, moodiness, and difficulty with mental cognitive skills.

Where Does Mercury Lurk?

As stated early, mercury is a common and naturally occurring element that is used in many different areas of our lives. It can be found in fish, shellfish, soil, water, and even in the air around us. It is also used in household items, thermometers, industrial products, and coal.

Amalgam Fillings

Many people are familiar with the silver fillings used here in the United States for the last century. Many dentists found them to be strong, cost effective, and durable. Unfortunately, the amalgam is a mercury compound composed of 50% elemental mercury and 50% a combination of other metals such as silver, tin, and copper. These fillings are regulated by the FDA and are considered safe for use by that agency. Both the Center for Disease Control (CDC) and the FDA have released information purporting the benefits of these fillings as safe and effective although the FDA did revise its recommendation, suggesting that pregnant women refrain from receiving these types fillings.

However, there is growing concern among the civilian scientific community regarding the mercury found in these fillings. Independent studies have shown that these types of fillings leach out harmful toxins into the body of the patient. According to a study conducted by the International Academy of Oral Medicine and Toxicology (IAOMT), these fillings release harmful vapors which will then find their way into the brain, blood stream, and later into the different organs and glands of the body. The amount of vapors released increases with normal activity such as chewing, grinding, with elevated body heat, or during other dental procedures.

Did You Know?

According to the IAOMT, the following are all symptoms of mercury exposure through amalgam fillings:

*Irritability	*Insomnia	*Anxiety	*Memory Loss
*Depression	*Drowsiness	*Concentration Difficulties	*Muscle Weakness
*Poor Balance	*Tremors	*Numbness in the Hands & Feet	*Bleeding Gums
*Headaches	*Stiff Neck	*Metallic Taste	*Speech Impairment
*Numbness in the Face	*Ringing in the Ears	*Nausea	*Burning in the Lips

Alternatives to amalgam fillings do exist and are gaining in popularity as more information becomes available to the public about the potential dangers of mercury poisoning. Such alternatives include resin composites, glass and resin ionomers, pure gold, and porcelain. If you are faced with future dental work that requires a filling, I strongly suggest talking to your dentist about one of these types of fillings instead of the traditional amalgam.

So what can you do if you already have amalgam fillings? First, visit the <u>American College of Advanced Medicine</u> (ACAM) to find a holistic practitioner in your area who can safely remove the fillings and replace them with a safe alternative. You will also need to speak to your physician about heavy metal detoxification to remove the mercury deposits already in your body.

> **Author's Note: For further information about heavy metal detoxification, I highly recommend Andrew Hall Cutler's Book *Amalgam Illness, Diagnosis and Treatment : What You Can Do to Get Better, How Your Doctor Can Help*. This book has helped me enormously and I recommend it to all my friends, family, and clients.**

Batteries

The vast majority of batteries used the America today do not contain any mercury. There is zero chance of exposure from the standard batteries you use in your remote controls, game controllers, or smoke detectors. There are two main exceptions to this rule are mercuric oxide batteries and button cell batteries.

Mercuric oxide batteries are used in the medical and emergency services fields due to the reliability of current and the extended lifespan of the batteries. These are essential qualities to have which are unmatched in non mercury batteries of comparable size. Button cell batteries are more common and more easily recognizable to most adults. These batteries are the small button shaped batteries commonly used in watches and small electronic devices.

There are no federal regulations regarding the use and disposal of button cell batteries. You can safely discard them in the garbage without incurring a federal infraction. They do not have to be labeled. Recycling of these items is very rare.

There is little data available regarding potential hazards of these batteries. As a precaution, you will not want to remain in an area where a battery of this nature has ruptured and any contaminates are leaking. Seek medical attention if you should become exposed to any of the chemicals on the inside of the battery. But don't allow yourself to worry about the possibility of exposure from this source. They are extremely safe.

Light Bulbs

Unlike incandescent light bulbs popular over the past century, fluorescent light bulbs use electricity to activate mercury vapors within the bulb or tube. These vapors heat up and create ultraviolet light.

Over the past few years, Compact Fluorescent Lights (CFL) have gained in popularity replacing the older incandescent bulbs. These CFLs are more energy efficient and cost effective. They are completely safe as long as they remain intact and unbroken.

Problems develop with the bulbs shatter or break. Remember they contain vaporized mercury which has been heated to create light. As we discussed above, this leads to a real potential for mercury poisoning through inhalation. If you are in any area with a broken CFL light bulb, leave the area immediately. According to the EPA, you should ventilate the area for at least 10 minutes before reentering; turn off the HVAC system to prevent further distribution of mercury vapors; then upon reentering carefully pick up the broken pieces of the light bulb using rubber gloves and disposal towels. Do not sweep or vacuum the area as this may cause more harmful vapors to circulate throughout the air. Continue to air the room for without running the HVAC system for several hours to ensure the vapors have completely disappeared.

Did You Know?

If one, only one, mercury thermometer breaks in a school, OSHA guidelines require the area to be evacuated and a specialized Hazmat team has to be sent in to clean up the spill! Yet many adults walk around with that much mercury in their mouths.

Maximize Your Safety around Toxins

As we've seen, toxins can be found in a number of locations and products commonly used in everyday life. These toxins can great affect your health and the quality of life you enjoy. Many of these items have been deemed safe for general use and can be beneficial.

However, you should always use proper precautions when dealing with a toxin to limit the risk of exposure. Doing so can save you lots of pain and suffering as well as a fair amount of money in future healthcare costs!

Mercury Poisoning and Me

Going to the dentist is never fun for anyone, especially if you have to go and get a filling for a cavity. For many of us born before the 1980s, this meant coming home with a silver looking substance in one of your back tooth. No fun, but no big deal either, right? Wrong!

Those silver looking fillings used for over a hundred years in the states are what are known as amalgam fillings, a combination of metals composed mainly of liquid mercury plus a mixture of silver, tin, and copper. They are still being used though not as widely, but in some other countries the use of amalgam fillings is banned.

As we just discussed, Mercury is highly toxic. Not a great combination to be putting into the bodies of millions of Americans!

After doing a fairly extensive amount of research, and by having specialized testing done, I discovered that I was also suffering from mercury poisoning which was directly associated and caused by the mercury in my metal fillings. I wanted to detox my body, but further research convinced me that the only way to effectively do that was by removing the source of the metal, then removing the deposits of metal throughout my body.

I was fortunate because at that time I only had two remaining amalgam fillings. I decided to have my fillings removed by the only dentists that can safely remove mercury from your mouth, an accredited dentist/member of the International Academy of Oral Medicine, and Toxicology (better known as IAOMT). I had my fillings removed on June 10, 2014 and it has definitely helped me. I am feeling much better. My food tastes better. And best of all, I can tell a marked difference in the level of anxiety that I suffer from. It was a completely worthwhile investment for me and one I hope you'll consider making for yourself.

Chapter 5 Diet & Exercise

"Let thy food be thy medicine and thy medicine be thy food." Hippocrates spoke these immortal words some 2,500 years ago. Unfortunately, it's a lesson we still have not fully learned today. In the most prosperous nation in the world, many people go without meeting the recommended daily allowances of many essential vitamins and minerals. An estimated 57% of the U.S. population does not meet the minimum dietary intake of magnesium, a leading contributor in anxiety disorders. We must give our bodies the fuels needed to heal ourselves from the inside out.

I learned this lesson the hard way. For many years, I avoided vegetables like the plague. And my body suffered dearly for that. I always thought that I was getting the necessary nutrients from my daily vitamins. I couldn't have been more wrong. As we'll see shortly, I damaged my body more than I could know and am now working to correct those issues.

There is no doubt that exercise plays a substantial role in physical fitness. It has long been proven that the more we move our bodies, the better our bodies will perform. But did you know, that exercise can greatly reduce the level of anxiety and stress you feel throughout the entire day?

As we mentioned in Chapter 4, exercise increases the release of endorphins into the body. These endorphins create an internal euphoria in the brain, a natural high. But unlike a chemically induced high, it takes the body more time to come down. The euphoria lasts longer creating a prolonged positive feeling after a workout. Studies suggest that people who exercise regularly are 25% less likely to experience anxiety and depression than those who don't.

Even a short burst of exercise will generate positive mental results. A quick 20 minute walk has been shown to produce the same anxiety reducing effects as a .25mg Xanax. While the shorter sessions will produce an immediate result, it will only be a temporary feeling as opposed to the long lasting effects of regular sustained exercise.

Incorporating Exercise into Therapy

Provided you are healthy enough to begin an exercise regime, exercising as a form of therapy is an excellent way to stabilize and improve mental health and cognitive skills. Research shows that it is equally as effective as meditation and may reduce the need for anti-anxiety medication.

As with all treatments, the benefits vary from person to person. Some individuals may see a drastic decrease in the level of anxiety while others may see only a moderate change. Likewise, not all forms of exercise work well for all people. Your best friend may be an avid runner, yet you detest the very idea of running unless you're being chased by a large, hungry animal. Walking or biking may be a better fit for you.

Don't be afraid to experiment with different types of exercise until you find several that you truly enjoy. Whether it be yoga, kick boxing, cycling, weight lifting, or swimming, the important thing is to get those endorphins flowing to help improve your mental health.

Tips & Tricks

To fully reap the benefits of therapeutic exercise, stick to a regular daily schedule. This will help prevent lapses that may derail your therapy all together. Write this time on your calendar. Consider it 'your' time. It's not a time for the kids, your spouse, work, or school. It's your personal time to unwind and decompress.

Start off slowly and build your way up to your goals. If you're completely sedentary now, start with a moderately easy exercise like walking. Plan to initially walk for 20 minutes a day, then, in a week or two, increase the amount of time you walk until you're walking 45 minutes to an hour each day. As your body begins to develop, incorporate new forms of exercise into your regimen. Try new things and create a routine that works for you.

Utilize distractions when necessary. Don't like walking for that long because it gives you too much time to think about stressors? Use your iPod to listen to music or an audio book while you walk. The distraction will prevent the negative thoughts from creeping in and help you pass the time. Better yet, find a friend to work out with and enjoy a tech free conversation with your bestie.

Finally, cut yourself a little slack. Your body will need time to adjust to your new found love of exercise, especially if you are currently a comfortable couch potato. Give yourself some time. Don't expect to run a marathon tomorrow. (Or a 5K either, for that matter.) It usually takes a month or two before your body truly acclimates to the routine. Don't give up after a few days. You can do it. I believe in you!

Your Diet and Anxiety

Just as exercise plays a major role in anxiety reduction, so too does diet. Your body needs specialized nutrients to produce the necessary hormones and neurotransmitters required for good mental health. The easiest way to get those nutrients is by modifying your diet to include foods that promote good mental health. There are numerous options to choose from.

For starters, pick complex carbohydrates over processed carbohydrates. Foods like oatmeal, quinoa, and whole grain breads increase the level of serotonin in your body. They breakdown slowly, so the calming effect is prolonged and will last for several hours. Avoid overly processed foods like white bread, sugary cereals, and sodas. They too are carbohydrates, but as we saw in the previous chapter, they do more harm to the body than good.

Eat a healthy breakfast with protein. Protein also breaks down slowly so you feel fuller for a longer period of time. Plus protein is essential in the production of neurotransmitters. You begin your day by stimulating the positive messengers in your brain.

Lastly, drink plenty of water. Your body needs water to function proper. After all, it is almost 70% water. Dehydration can greatly alter mood and make cognitive processes difficult at best. Switching from sugary and caffeinated drinks to water will greatly improve your mental facilities.

Almonds

Almonds and other nuts contain B complex vitamins as well as a host of minerals such as magnesium and calcium which have been shown to greatly improve mental health.

Magnesium deficiency has been shown in many studies to produce anxiety and depression in patients. As the fourth most abundant mineral in our bodies, it plays a major role in many areas of our lives. Magnesium supplements are often prescribed to relieve constipation. Yet it also affects our kidneys, helps prevent diabetes, and reduces the likelihood of osteoporosis. Common side effects of magnesium deficiency are anxiety, low energy, headaches, fatigue, and muscle cramping.

If you remember our discussion in Chapter 2 regarding the parathyroid, you know calcium acts as the conductor of electric currents in the nervous system. But is also works with the body to ensure proper magnesium absorption. By maintaining a proper level of calcium in the body, your body will be better able to process magnesium.

And almonds pack a powerful magnesium/calcium punch. Each almond contains approximately 3mg of each mineral. Unlike other nuts, the calcium-magnesium ratio in almonds is 1-1. It's difficult to beat that combination.

Did You Know?

Two handfuls of cashews offer the same depression and anxiety relief as a prescription dose of Prozac!

Beef

Red meat such as beef is an excellent source of iron, B vitamins, zinc, and proteins necessary for muscle and organ development. Studies conducted in Deakin University in Melbourne, Australia shows a direct link between the increase in anxiety, depression, and other mood disorders with a reduced intake in red meat. They studied 1000 women to determine the effects of red meat on mood disorders. Their results were not exactly what they expected.

> "We had originally thought that red meat might not be good for mental health, as studies from other countries had found red meat consumption to be associated with physical health risks, but it turns out that it actually may be quite important," said Felice Jacka, Ph.D., associate professor from Deakin's Barwon Psychiatric Research Unit.
>
> "When we looked at women consuming less than the recommended amount of red meat in our study, we found that they were twice as likely to have a diagnosed depressive or anxiety disorder as those consuming the recommended amount," she said. (Pederson, 2012)

They also found that proteins found in other meats such as chicken, fish, and pork and plant based proteins did not have the same benefits for mental health. As their study strongly suggests, red meat consumption helps improve mental health.

That's not to say there are not health factors to consider when adding red meat to your diet. It has been shown to increase the risk of certain types of cancers, increase cholesterol levels, and lead to weight gain. Therefore, you should always consume red meat in moderation.

Red meat should not be the main staple of protein in your diet. It should be eaten occasionally instead of daily. Recommended allowances of red meat suggest no more than 17 ounces per week. That is approximately three small steaks per week. When choosing the types of red meat to eat, pick a cut that is lean and lower in overall fat content as that will help reduce the other risk factors. If possible, it is best to choose grass-fed beef.

Beef and lamb are excellent sources of mood enhancing proteins, minerals, and vitamins. They can definitely lower your overall levels of anxiety if eaten in moderation.

Did You Know?

You can order grass-fed organic meats from www.grasslandbeef.com. Best of all, they bring if right to your door!

Blueberries

Blueberries are nature's wonder berry. They contain a plethora of antioxidants. In fact they have the highest antioxidant concentration of all fruits. They have been used around the world to fight a wide variety of conditions such as digestive issues, promote urinary tract health, improve vision, and reduce belly fat.

And, they are extremely beneficial in reducing the levels of anxiety and depression. In addition to antioxidants, blueberries are high in vitamin C. In fact, just one cup of fresh blueberries has one fourth of the recommended daily allowance of vitamin C. Why is vitamin C important? Because it reduces blood pressure and helps keep cortisol level in check. By reducing a major symptom (elevated blood pressure) and regulating the master stress hormone, blueberries provide a two prong assault on anxiety.

Interestingly enough, some experts believe that blueberries can protect against brain damage caused by toxins. As we learned in Chapter 4, toxins can wreak havoc on your brain and the neurotransmitters that function there. The antioxidants in blueberries have been shown to slow the progress of the degeneration.

As you can see, blueberries are the wonder fruit of nature. Not only are they beneficial for your overall health but they provide a great source of anxiety fighting vitamins that will help you alleviate anxiety for good!

Chocolate

Great news for chocoholics everywhere! Studies have shown that chocolate can help reduce stress and anxiety. This doesn't mean indulge in the jumbo bag of M&M's or grab the nearest milk chocolate bar. The type of chocolate we're referring to here is dark chocolate without a lot of processed sugars. The chocolate should contain 70% cacao or more.

So how does chocolate affect mood? There are several theories to that question that have yet to be answered completely but many scientists believe that it increases the production of serotonin in the brain. As we learned in Chapter 3, serotonin is a vital component in determining mood.

Another possible reason for chocolate's mood enhancing qualities is its main ingredient, Theobromine. Studies seem to suggest this chemical is directly linked mood elevation when ingested. Chocolate contains large amounts of magnesium which helps fight anxiety.

The research on chocolate as an anxiety fighter still needs to be expanded on. However, based on preliminary findings, a piece of dark chocolate could be a welcome addition in your anxiety fighting arsenal. Keep in mind though that you shouldn't try to fight anxiety solely by eating chocolate! A balanced diet incorporating the foods we've mentioned here is a far better solution than that. But, when eaten in moderation, chocolate can make you feel better, as so many chocolate lovers can attest to!

Salmon

It may seem strange that I would include salmon as among the anti-anxiety foods to eat after addressing the concerns of mercury poisoning in the previous chapter, but salmon and other types of fish offer our bodies an excellent source of Omega-3 fatty acids.

So what exactly is Omega3? Omega 3s are the good type of fat that your body needs to maximize health. They help remove fatty deposits from your blood, relieve stiffness in joints, fight depression and Alzheimer's disease, and reduce the risk of asthma attacks.

Salmon contains a high concentration of Omega 3 (wild contains more than farmed), but other types of fish are also high in this essential fat such as lake trout, herring, and tuna. All are good sources to incorporate into your diet. To avoid fish with a higher mercury content, try to stay away from shark, mackerel, and swordfish as these have all been shown to contain high levels of mercury and other toxins.

Soy

There is still a lot of uncertainty about the full benefits of soy. Some studies suggest that soy offers the most mental health benefits in men and women who are premenstrual. It has also been shown to help alleviate menopausal symptoms such as hot flashes and night sweats in women.

Most experts agree that soy helps improve cognitive function and reduces the risk of osteoporosis. It also appears that soy plays a substantial role in heart health. Lastly, it has been linked to the reduced risk of some forms of cancer.

Experts agree that soy can be beneficial in numerous ways including fighting depression and reducing anxiety. This is believed to be a direct result from the isoflavones so abundant in soy beans.

To maximize the potential benefit of soy and isoflavones, consume only natural forms of soy such as whole soy beans or edamame in salads. Avoid processed forms of soy products as these will often contain added sugars and will reduce the efficiency of absorption.

Turkey

We learned in Chapter 2 that turkey is a great source of melatonin, the hormone responsible for sleep regulation. You probably know this already from your experiences with a large Thanksgiving dinner. Turkey will make you sleepy.

But turkey also contains a substance called tryptophan which is essential in the production of serotonin. The higher the level of tryptophan your body maintains the more serotonin it will be able to efficiently produce.

Balanced Nutrition and Exercise

As you can see, diet and exercise go hand in hand with the promotion of positive mental health. These changes don't happen overnight, especially if you suffer from any of the food additions we will discuss in Chapter 6! It will take time for your body to detox from those harmful foods.

Additionally, you should be sensitive to any food allergies you may have. We will discuss those in more detail in Chapter 7. Listen to your body to create the anxiety reducing diet that works for you.

Finally, incorporate exercise into your life in a slow but steady manner. You are not competing with anyone else here. You are trying to make your body and mind the best you can be. You're trying to improve your quality of life. Experiment until you find what works for you and stick with it.

> **Beware of Over Exercising!**
>
> I have been an avid fitness enthusiast since my early teens. I mean when other girls were playing with make-up, I was lifting weights at home. For me, it's a passion that has developed into a way of life. Personally, in the past I would have never imagined

not going to the gym to workout. Unfortunately, I learned the hard way that too much of a good thing can be detrimental.

I actively competed in figure competitions from 2007 until 2012. That lifestyle involves a lot of intense training and a very strict diet, all this to help sculpt and perfect your muscle tone and decrease your body's fat content. For each show I would get my body fat down and under 10%. And during the off season my body fat would stay around 13%, which was very unhealthy. Now I don't mention this to brag, actually I am a very humble and modest person, I just tell you this to paint a picture of how avid of a gym rat I was and how unhealthy I was living.

Just to paint a clearer picture, the average 19-29 year old American women's body fat range is between 23-25% and mine was 13% during off season. I was trying to maintain a life that was unrealistic!

When I would prepare for a competition, I was very mindful of everything I put into my mouth. I wouldn't drink anything other than water and possibly decaf coffee (without the cream of course). For the 12 weeks it took to prepare leading up to a show I wouldn't cheat at all. I was determined to be the best I could be.

Or at least I thought that would make me the best I could be. Little did I know my decision to compete and therefore deplete myself of the fat and nutrients my body so desperately needed attributed to my many hormonal imbalances, including those of my thyroid and adrenals.

The good news is I walked away with several trophies and I can gloat that I accomplished a childhood dream, but the bad news is I now have to clean up the mess it caused inside my body.

You see, one of my major problems back then, was the fact that I didn't like vegetables. I wasn't concerned with what it would do inside my body if I didn't eat them. I mean I was taking a multi-vitamin so I should have been ok, right? Wrong! As a result, my diet was far from balanced. At that time I didn't eat fresh salads and greens, like I do today, I was focused on my workouts and I didn't give any thought to how important greens were. As my caloric intake decreased, a lot of the essential vitamins and minerals my body needed went with it. Add to that the fact that I was performing hours of strenuous physical routines per week and it put a severe strain on my hormones, most importantly my thyroid and adrenals.

I've since stopped competing and have since introduced lots of fruits and vegetables into my diet. And now I LOVE them! I even completed my Health Coaching certification from the Institute for Integrative Nutrition and now my husband referrers to me as a "Health Nut," all joking aside as a result to my new lifestyle, I'm much healthier now than I was when I was in competition form. So many people get it wrong and look up to those competing thinking they're the picture of health, but actually if you could see them from the inside you would realize that is far

> from the truth.
>
> Getting my hormones (progesterone, thyroid and adrenals) under control and removing benzos from my life greatly improved my mental state. Now I can reap the mental benefits of exercise, that runner's high, which for so long was elusive.

Pederson, T. (2012, 03 21). *Not Enough Red Meat Tied to Anxiety and Depression in Women.* Retrieved from Psych Central: http://psychcentral.com/news/2012/03/21/women-eat-red-meat-to-lessen-anxiety-depression/36348.html

Chapter 6 Addiction & Dependency

When most people hear the word addiction they immediately think about lawless drug cartels or street level thugs. But addiction does not necessarily encompass those aspects of society. Many people in our society today suffer from some form of dependency although they don't readily recognize the signs and symptoms.

Webster's defines addiction this way, "A strong and harmful need to regularly have something (such as a drug) or do something (such as gamble)." While its definition of dependence is, "The state of being physically or psychologically dependent; addiction." Even though the two words are synonymous, most people the word dependency because it tends to be less judgmental. I am one of them. Having suffered from dependency on benzodiazepine, I know firsthand how easy it is for your body to become dependent on a substance and how difficult it is to rid your body of that substance.

Regardless of the substance or habit in question, dependency is hard to break!

But, it's not impossible. The first step is to recognize that your body is dependent and take steps to address the dependency head on. Remember as you start this journey, it will usually take your body four weeks to create a new habit. It may take longer depending on the strength of the dependency. Stick with it and don't get discouraged. You can rid your body of the harmful substances that are causing your anxiety for good.

It took me two years to break my dependency on benzos!! I know exactly how difficult that journey is because

I've walked that path myself. It was an uncomfortable truth I was faced with when I realized my body was dependent on that medication. I wasn't a path I wanted to venture down. Yet, freeing my body from its dependency has been an incredibly rewarding experience. It's a challenge I'm glad I accepted.

Alcohol

For many people social drinking is a great way to blow off steam and relax with friends and colleagues. Most scientists agree that moderate drinking does no harm to the body. However, it is often difficult for an individual to determine when alcohol consumption goes from moderate drinking to a fully fledged problem. It is a sneaky problem that takes many people and families by surprise although the signs were there from the beginning.

Alcohol is a depressant. It interferes with the neurotransmitters in the brain, directly affecting mood and behavior. It attacks the liver causing fatty deposits to collect which may develop into fibrosis or cirrhosis. It damages the heart and has been shown to increase blood pressure, cause arrhythmias, cardiomyopathy, and strokes. It attacks the pancreas and may lead to pancreatitis or insulin problems. Lastly, it is a known cause of several types of cancers.

It is possible to be what many people consider a social drinking and still have a drinking problem. If you find yourself hiding the amount of alcohol you consume from family and friends, ever feel guilty about drinking, or need a drink to relax then you may have an alcohol problem that needs monitoring.

So what is considered moderate drinking and how do you know if you're drinking too much? For women, doctors have determined that one drink per day is usually safe. A glass of wine during dinner or a beer during the big game is fine. Women who on average consume more than seven drinks per week or more than three drinks in a single sitting may be headed for a problem. For men, those numbers are generally doubled, two drinks per day but no more than four drinks in a single sitting or fourteen drinks in a week.

Alcohol Abuse

Alcohol abuse is different from alcoholism in that abusers have the ability to set limits on their alcohol consumption. This ability may be short-lived if external factors cause an onset of stress which may push the abuser into the realm of fully blown alcoholism.

That being said, alcohol does still negatively impact the daily lives of abusers. They may skip out on responsibilities such as work or school due to drinking issues. They may begin to mix alcohol with prescription medication or face legal consequences for driving under the influence of alcohol. They may use alcohol as a coping mechanism, to relieve stress from the day. They will often continue to consume alcohol even though it is causing problems with relationships.

There is no way of knowing if alcohol abuse will develop into true alcoholism. Some individuals seek out counseling and support groups for help. Others may have the support of family and friends to help reduce the level of alcohol consumed. However, alcohol abuse is a major risk factor for alcoholism. As one's tolerance level increases, so too does the amount of alcohol consumed. It is quite possible for an abuser to develop alcoholism without realizing the situation.

Alcoholism

Alcohol is a chronic condition which requires professional help to overcome. The first major sign of alcoholism is tolerance. As stated above, tolerance means that more alcohol is needed over time to get the same effects. This is the first sign of dependency.

Alcoholics face physical symptoms of withdrawal unlike those who abuse alcohol. Withdrawal symptoms include uncontrollable shaking, anxiety, sweating, nausea, vomiting, fatigue, irritability and moodiness, loss of appetite and headaches. Those who are dependent on alcohol will often drink to relieve these symptoms rather than face the pains of withdrawals. Some alcoholics go to great lengths to get alcohol if family and friends have attempted to create a dry environment. They may consume cold medicine or other products that contain alcohol. They may hide alcohol so that no one knows they are still drinking. They may blatantly leave home to go out on a bender.

People with this condition live in a state of denial. They rationalize their need for alcohol and mitigate the negative consequences. In order to correct the problem they will first have to admit the problem exists then seek professional help to overcome the addiction.

Did You Know?

Over 95% of all alcoholics are also hypoglycemic. Incorporating the supplement L-glutamine into their

> daily diets has been proven to regulate blood sugar swings and reduce the craving for alcohol sugars.

Caffeine

There is a lot of debate about caffeine addiction within the medical community due primarily to the medical definition of addiction which is a bit narrower than the definition we used above. However, for our purposes here, scientists do know that people can develop a habitual need for caffeine and will suffer from withdrawals if that need is not met.

Caffeine is most commonly found in tea leave and coffee beans. It is also present in cocoa beans, cough syrups, energy drinks, and sodas. You may be surprised at how much caffeine you are actually consuming in a day. Doctors recommend no more than 400mg of caffeine daily for most adults, or the equivalent of four cups of coffee. That number is reduced to 100mg in children and teens. These numbers are deemed safe but are generalized for the whole of society. You may be more or less tolerant of caffeine depending on the amount you normally consume, body mass, health conditions, age, and medications you are currently taking.

For some people, even one caffeinated drink causes an uneasy, jittery feeling and sleep loss while others who have developed a tolerance can drink caffeinated beverages throughout the day with little problems.

However, it is not a good idea to routinely consume large amounts of caffeine as it can cause side effects such as rapid heartbeat, irritability, insomnia, restlessness, muscle tremors, and stomach discomfort. If you routinely drink more than the recommended daily dose of caffeine or have experienced any of these signs, your body may be dependent on caffeine.

Caffeine dependency does cause physical symptoms including severe headaches that radiate through the head, drowsiness, difficulty concentrating or mental fuzziness, and flu like symptoms including aches and pains, nausea, and vomiting. The severity of the withdrawal symptoms will greatly depend on how dependent your body has become to caffeine. Your doctor may be able to give you medication which will alleviate some of these symptoms.

Did You Know?

Coffee has been shown to reduce blood circulation to the brain by 23%. This lack of circulation to the brain is a major contributing factor to anxiety.

Food Addiction

As we saw in Chapter 5, diet can play a major role in your body's response to stress as well as the production of anxiety reducing hormones. Unfortunately, it can also have the opposite effect if you consume the wrong types of foods as a normal part of your diet.

It may seem strange to list foods among a chapter dealing with addiction and dependency. Yet, each year, more and more people find out their bodies have become dependent on substances commonly found in the foods they eat. These dependencies are often difficult to break, with side effects that can rival other addictions. Your body craves these substances even though they have adverse overall effects. Your body only recognizes the immediate pleasure responses they create. Fortunately, you can overcome an addiction to food. It may seem difficult, but it is possible. Remember, it only takes four weeks to form a new habit.

Food addition has several tell-tell signs that you may have encountered in the past. Symptoms may include the inability to control cravings, feeling ashamed of weight or physical appearance, hiding the amount of food you eat, trying numerous different fad diet pills to enhance appearance, avoiding social interactions in which food is involved for fear that you won't be able to control your urges, eating as a reward, eating to deal with stress, and eating when you're not hungry. If you have experienced several of these symptoms, you may have an underlying problem with food addiction.

Sugar

Many people know the allure of sugar. We put it in coffee, tea, on cereal, and in many recipes that we make for our families. It can be found in sodas, cookies, ice cream, and deserts of all shapes and sizes. What most people don't realize is that it is also in items like ketchup, teriyaki sauce, and 'healthy' foods like yogurt and instant oatmeal. In this day and age, sugar literally is everywhere you look, although in many cases it's disguised.

According to the American Heart Association (AHA), adults should consume no more than six to nine teaspoons of sugar per day. That's 100 to 150 calories from sugar per day. However, by conservative estimates, we as a society are consuming ten times that amount daily. The average adult American eats about 132 pounds of sugar every year. 132 pounds! That's the size of a small adult. It takes 3500 calories to make a pound. When you calculate that, it's over 1200 calories per day in sugar.

Granted most people don't eat 1200 calories of sugar on a daily basis. You may go several days or a week with limited sugar intake. (By limited, I mean you watch what you eat and try to stay away from sweets and sodas.) Then you have a particularly stressful day, or a good day for that matter, and you crave a giant banana split or slab of cake. Wash that down with a soda or sweet drink and you've just drastically increased your sugar intake for the week.

But why do so many people crave sugar so desperately? For one thing, it makes food taste good. If that's all it did, then we'd be able to easily set it aside and moderate the levels we eat. However, it does much more than that. When we eat sugars or large amounts of processed carbohydrates such as breads or sugary cereals, it triggers our brains to release serotonin. As we learned in Chapter 3, serotonin creates a euphoric feeling in the brain. We feel happy for a few minutes or hours afterward. This sugar high is short lived and once it's over, our bodies' crash. We begin to feel fatigued.

Have you ever had a case of mid-afternoon blahs? You may have felt drowsy, tired, depressed, and a little out of it mentally. Then you eat a candy bar and for the next hour or so you're alert and productive only to fall harder after the effects wear off. The sugar in that candy bar has caused your body to receive a temporary sugar high. Once it's over, it's over and you crash. Hard.

There are physical consequences to sugar addiction as well. In addition to the bulging waist line and snug fitting clothing, people who regularly consume a large amount of sugar are more likely to develop Type 2 diabetes, heart disease, depression, gout, migraines, and arthritis.

To begin ridding your diet or sugar, take a close look at the ingredients on the packaging labels for your food. Chances are you'll see sugar, or type of sugar, somewhere in the mix. Also read the nutritional information listed. How many grams of sugar are listed?

Did You Know?

Sugar can be lurking anywhere in the ingredients list and is often disguised by different names. These different names tend to be from highly processed sugar products which are actually worse than natural sugar.

Don't be fooled! If you see any of these ingredients, you are looking at a highly processed sugar product.

Agave nectar	Corn syrup solids
Agave syrup	Crystalized fructose
Barley malt	Date sugar
Beet sugar	Dextran
Brown rice syrup	Dextrose
Brown sugar	Diatase
Buttered syrup	Diastatic malt
Cane sugar	Evaporated cane juice

Cane juice	Fructose	Ma
Cane juice crystals	Fruit juice	Mo
Carob syrup	Fruit juice concentrate	Raw
Confectioner's sugar	Glucose	Ref
Corn syrup	Glucose solids	Sor
High fructose corn syrup	Golden sugar	Suc
Corn sugar	Golden syrup	Suc
Corn sweetener	Grape sugar	Sug
		Tur
		Yel

Once you have found the hidden sources of sugar in your diet, begin eliminating them. Switch to fresh fruits and vegetables. Fruits are loaded in fiber which slows the absorption of fructose, the main sugar in all fruits, to the body. I recommend shopping only in the perimeter of the supermarket. That is where the least processed foods are. Switch from white bread to whole wheat bread instead. An even better option is to eliminate bread completely from your diet. Pack a healthy snack for your mid-afternoon energy crash, like an organic apple or handful of almonds.

Keep a journal of the foods you eat for several weeks and how you felt throughout the day. Did you have the same problem with energy crashes? Did you feel hungrier or fuller? Did you suffer from as many migraines? What about your emotional health? Were you as depressed or anxious? By keeping track of these things you can begin to see the actual affects sugar, or the lack thereof, has on your physical and emotional health. And once you've conquered your sugar addiction, you'll be less tempted to cave into that craving for ice cream that your friends can't seem to overcome.

Fatty Foods

Just like food with high quantities of sugars and processed sugars, fatty foods have one major flaw. They tend to taste great! Unfortunately, it's that great taste that may lure you in and begin a journey into fatty food addiction.

Many scientists now believe that the addiction and dependency to fatty foods may be as difficult to break as cocaine addiction. When we eat foods with a high fat content, our bodies trigger the production and release of dopamine. We learned about this neurotransmitter in Chapter 3. Like the serotonin released while eating sugary foods, the dopamine produces an instant, natural high within the body. You feel happy and euphoric. But this high is short lived and eventually, it will take more and more of the same foods to elicit the same response.

Unfortunately, many of the foods you are probably eating now contain both high quantities of fat and sugar, so it becomes a double edged sword. You may not begin to see the results you want, and to feel better on an emotional level, until you address both fatty and sugary foods in your diet.

Now you realize that you cannot cut all fats out of your diet. It's dangerous and you shouldn't try to. Your brain needs fat to function properly. It just doesn't need excessive amounts of fat. The AHA recommends no more than 30% of your daily diet come from fatty foods, or roughly 65 grams of fat for a 2,000 calorie per day diet. If you eat at a fast food restaurant once a day, you have just exceeded that limit even if you eat healthy the rest of the day. Anything more may adversely affect your body's ability to fight off cravings.

Salt

According to studies conducted at Duke University and the University of Melbourne, sodium activates the same neurotransmitters as highly addictive drugs do. This leads credence to what many people are calling salt addiction and may explain why so many people experience intense salt cravings.

The major difference between salt and addictive drugs is that our bodies need some salt to properly function. It's a similar situation to fatty foods which we just spoke about. Our bodies need salt but we need it in moderation.

The recommended daily allowance for salt and sodium intake is 1500mg. However, there are many people who routinely consume far more than that amount. Sometimes they consume as much as five times that amount. And they may not even know how much salt they are eating.

Most of the salt Americans consume comes from packaged and processed foods. One single serving of a frozen dinner can contain as much as 800 or 900mg of sodium. In one meal, you could easily consume 2/3 the recommended daily allowance. That doesn't begin to account for all the hidden sodium in much of the food we eat!

People who routinely consume excessive amounts of salt are at risk for numerous health conditions. They may develop high blood pressure and have water retention. This is a dangerous combination as excess fluid can often settle on the lungs, heart, or other internal organs. Additionally, they may experience changes in urination and uncontrollable thirst.

To reduce the level of salt intake, cut out processed foods that contain massive amounts of sodium. Avoid foods with visible amounts of salt such as pretzels and chips. Leave the salt shaker in the kitchen and off the table. Experiment with other spices to add flavor to foods without the added sodium. Limit condiments such as ketchup, dressings, and soy sauce. With a little effort, you can easily get your sodium intake under control.

Illegal Drugs

For the purposes of this book, we will not delve extensively into the world of illegal drugs. It is important to note, if you are taking any form of illegal drugs, even for recreational purposes, you are contributing to your anxiety problems. Amphetamines, cocaine, LSD, and ecstasy have all been shown to cause anxiety, rapid heartbeats, panic attacks, or hallucinations. These effects increase dramatically when illegal drugs are combined with one another or with alcohol.

It is unclear whether the long term effects of illegal drug use are responsible for prolonged periods of anxiety after a patient is successfully weaned off the drug. It may be that the narcotic changed in brain function drastically alter the neurotransmitters and thereby interfere with proper hormone regulation. However, one thing is clear, illegal drugs have a long history of causing anxiety and panic in users. If you are serious about reducing anxiety, say nope to dope!

Marijuana

There is currently much debate about the legalization of marijuana here in the country. Some states, like Colorado and Washington, have legalized marijuana for recreational use. As of this writing, 21 states in total plus the District of Columbia have legalized medical marijuana. We will not be passing judgment on these legal developments but we will discuss the relationship between marijuana and anxiety.

As difficult as it may be for most people to believe, marijuana has been shown to increase or induce panic in users. Although many people use marijuana to relax or calm down, it appears it may have adverse effects on anxiety particularly if the user suffers from a severe form of anxiety. Keep in mind these tests have been conducted in the safety of scientific labs under controlled environments. They were not using street level marijuana from a local dealer. Street marijuana is often laced with chemicals and additives which greatly alter the effects normally seen.

The studies conducted showed that the severity of the reaction was related to the type of anxiety suffered by the user. Anxiety that is compounded by negative thoughts is often amplified by marijuana use. It seems the drug does not change the overall mood; it only heightens the mood itself. A person suffering from anxiety will experience elevated levels of anxiety while a person who doesn't suffer from anxiety and depression may suffer few mood altering side effects.

The best bet if you are trying to lessen your anxiety is to stir clear of marijuana. While there may be some medical benefits (again, we're not going to address those here!), in the world of anxiety treatments, it will only worsen the problem.

Prescription Medication

Dependency on prescription medication comes in two distinctive categories, those who take the drugs by choice, often illegally, and those who become addicted while under medical supervision.

Many people first encounter prescription medication through recreational drug use at parties or through friends. If you are, or know someone who is taking prescription medication in this manner, you are in violation of the law. It is no different than any other form of illegal drug. Taking prescription drugs that were prescribed for someone else, or worse, randomly sold on the street is exceedingly dangerous. You should get help now.

The other group is the people who have become dependent on prescription medication while under the care of a physician. It may seem strange that dependency and addiction can occur while under the supervision of a doctor, but in many cases that does happen. Medications, particularly those that are used to treat pain, anxiety, and ADHD, can alter the chemical production in the brain. Over time, these changes create a dependency on the medication. It may be impossible for the patient to cease using the medication without the assistance of a trained addiction specialist.

Adderall and Ritalin

The two most commonly prescribed medications for ADHD affect the brain in similar ways. They both target the production and absorption of dopamine in the brain. And they both work by increasing the secretion of dopamine. Finally, they both contain an amphetamine stimulant which makes them very desirable for street level distribution.

Signs of addiction may include heart palpitations and fluctuations, nervousness, weight loss, headaches, paranoia, violent behavior, and seizures. The withdrawal symptoms can be equally severe. Most patients experience depression or anxiety, insomnia, excessive sweating, or lethargy. Addiction to these types of medications are serious and treatment should not be attempted without a trained medical professional to monitor the condition of the patient as their body recovers from the withdrawal pains.

Benzodiazepines

It is an unfortunate truth that the very medication you're taking to relieve your anxiety may actually be causing an increase in your anxiety. Benzodiazepines, or benzos, for short, are considered a safe drug for patients to use especially when treating conditions such an insomnia and anxiety on an as needed basis. This common conception often means that physicians with little or no psychiatric training feel confident in prescribing the medication to patients.

Therein lies a major part of the problem. These drugs are often being prescribed for individuals with long-term anxiety that should be on another form of medication not designed for an as needed use. These drugs were not designed to be a long-term solution. As a result, the brain becomes dependent on the medication to regulate anxiety hormones and neurotransmitters. The body will develop a tolerance over time requiring more and more of the medication to reap the same benefits. Thus it becomes a never ending cycle.

Patients who have taken benzos for a relatively long time, for example six months or more often experience severe side effects to stopping the medication. These side effects include increased panic and anxiety attacks, depression, rapid heartbeat, detachment or depersonalization, an inability to emote, delusions, psychosis, and tremors. These symptoms may be present in some patients for up to two years after successfully stopping the medication. Patients should not stop taking this medication suddenly as one or multiple symptoms may occur. Instead, seek out a medical professional training in benzo addiction to begin tapering off the medication for good.

Did You Know?

Benzos should never be taken for more than two consecutive weeks. In that short amount of time, your body can develop a dependency in some manner.

Opioids

Derived from the poppy plants, opioids are primarily used for pain relief. They work in much the same way, creating a feeling of euphoria in the patients. Opioids also inhibit the pain receptors in the body. For anyone who has been in considerable pain for an extended period of time, the feeling can be unlike anything they've ever felt before.

Symptoms of opioid addiction include weight loss, loss of appetite, paranoia, headaches, anxiety, confusion, forgetfulness, mood swings, and social isolation. Suffers may neglect family and friends, they may neglect personal hygiene, and may act irrationally such as selling off personal property or making illogical decisions.

Opioid addiction is a serious medical condition with painful withdrawal symptoms for those who wish to get help. It is vital therefore to contact a medical professional with experience in drug addiction before attempting to stop the dependency.

Tobacco

Tobacco and nicotine addiction are the most prevalent and preventable cause of death in the United States. Approximately one out of every 5 deaths is a direct result of tobacco use. What's more, tobacco use affects millions of nonsmokers who suffer adverse effects of secondhand smoke.

When you smoke or chew tobacco, nicotine enters the blood stream and stimulates the adrenal gland to release adrenaline. This rapid release of adrenaline increases blood pressure and heart rate almost immediately. It also works like other drugs such as cocaine to increase the release of dopamine giving the smoker a instant high. As we've seen before, this helps create the addiction of the substance.

Once a smoker becomes dependent on tobacco, it is difficult to quit. He may face severe withdrawal symptoms such as mood swings and irritability, difficulty concentrating, sleep disturbances, and a drastic increase in appetite. However, it is essential that smoker's make every effort to quit, not only for good mental health but for physical health as well.

Dependency and Emotional Well-being

As you can see, dependency on any substance can greatly alter your chemical and hormonal balance. Even substances that our bodies need on a daily basis like salt and fatty foods can become detrimental if consumed in excess. Once your hormonal harmony has been disrupted, it is difficult, but not impossible to realign.

It takes determination, will power, and commitment to overcome dependency on any substance. But the results are well worth the effort. Once your body is free from all the negative substances you've been putting in it for years, you'll be amazed at how much better you feel and how positive the affect will be on your emotional well-being.

My Benzo Dependency

My story into benzo dependency started like many others. I began taking Xanax (on a need to basis), a well known benzo around 1998 or 1999 while I was away at college. I was young, away from home, and living an unhealthy lifestyle. My doctor prescribed the medication at first to help me sleep and it work wonderfully, that was until I needed more of it. As a young college student, I trusted my doctor and thought everything was fine.

I remained on that medication, occasionally taking other anti-anxiety medications as recommended of my physician. I noticed after a while of taking the medication at night for sleep grew to me needing to take it during the day for anxiety. And the longer I took it, the more I needed it, and the each time the symptoms would become worse and so the dosage needed to be increased. Fortunately, I had the wherewithal to stop taking those medications during both of my pregnancies. I'm truly thankful that I didn't inadvertently pass any type of dependency onto my unborn children.

The withdrawal symptoms were extreme, but I believed it was complications with pregnancy or stress from work.

I remained on that medication for almost 15 years, and then finally in 2012, I made the decision to clean my body of this drug once and for all. It was a tough decision to make but one I felt was right for me. If the decision was difficult, the actually implementation of that decision was excruciating. In February 2012, I went to an outpatient detox center to help taper off the benzos for good. They switch me from Xanax (a fast acting benzo) to Valium (a slower acting benzo that stays in your body longer) to help ease the symptoms of withdrawal, but they attempted to take me off the benzos altogether too quickly.

As luck would have it, I switched jobs in May 2012, changing insurance companies in the process, which was a blessing from heaven because I was forced to find a new physician. That's when the doctor revealed to me that I was in a somewhat dangerous situation, I was in benzo withdrawal and therefore he tweaked my benzo dosage and suggested I add another medication to help me taper off the rest of the benzos, that drug was Remeron. I did as the doctor recommended and eventually after withdraw ling from the benzo I then had to withdrawal off Remeron, which was another gut wrenching experience, but I won't go into details on that in this book.

During my withdrawal of benzos I had

gastrointestinal issues, so I sought the help from a GI doctor. He and I spoke at lengths and I told him the journey I was on and he said this to me, "You have to find what's causing you to be anxious." And so began my quest for knowledge and the inspiration for this book. It's been a long journey, over two years in the making, but I can say, I am free and clean of benzos for good. The process was painful, costly, and emotionally draining, but I haven't felt better in years and I have no doubt this is just the beginning!

Just to relay how difficult detoxing from a benzo can be. They say it's harder to come off a benzo than it is to come off of heroin. The physical side effects of heroin detox may last a few weeks, but the physical and psychological side effects of coming off a benzo can last for YEARS. Please steer clear of this drug at all costs. I understand there are real medical needs for this drug like during surgery and during child birth, but it shouldn't be taken on an as need basis because that too will cause dependency and soon your anxiety will increase because of it.

Find the root cause of your anxiety

Chapter 7 Allergens & the Environment

Scientists are still learning about the complex relationship between allergies and anxiety. Part of the problem is individuality. Every person responds differently to different allergens. What may cause mild irritation to one person can be potentially life threatening to another. As we've mentioned before, the same is true of anxiety and depression. Therefore, it makes finding the common denominator fairly difficult.

What is known about allergies is that they can alter brain and body functions. These changes can trigger an anxiety episode. People who suffer from allergies generally tend to feel worse than those who don't which can lead to depression and anxiety. No allergens have been shown to directly cause anxiety, but they do seem to heighten the sensation.

Likewise, anxiety has a direct effect on allergy attacks. Anxiety won't cause you to develop an allergy but if you suffer from allergies, you will experience a stronger allergy attack with anxiety.

One common theory among experts is that allergens cause direct and indirect stress. You feel worse during an allergic reaction than when you're perfectly healthy. Experts theorize that it may be this stress that brings on the anxiety episode in sufferers.

More research must be done in this area, especially in the area of food allergies. As we learned in Chapter 5, what we put in our bodies directly affects the moods we feel. Eliminating an entire food or food category greatly affects which nutrients our body has to work with. And if we're missing too many essential nutrients, our bodies will spiral out of control.

But we must also monitor what we put on our bodies. Many of the health and beauty products most people normally use are laden with chemicals and allergens. That's why I decided to incorporate natural solutions into my daily beauty routine. I use coconut oil as a makeup remover and a full body lotion. I use natural hair soap and unfiltered apple cider vinegar as conditioner. The vinegar is well suited for balancing pH levels both internally and externally. It also works well as a facial toner. Avocado oil has become my favorite moisturizer! I use aluminum-free deodorant, use fluoride-free toothpaste, and all natural. People are regularly telling me I look younger than my age even though I do not spend a dime on the fancy name brand cosmetic lines.

Removing allergens from your life and the lives of your family can happen, but it takes some planning and initiative on your part. You'll be amazed at the results once you take that step forward.

Food Allergens

An estimated 220 to 520 million people worldwide are affected with some form of food allergy. Many of those sufferers are children under the age of 18. Over 12 million people in the United States alone have been diagnosed with a food allergy. Many more sufferers have never been diagnosed. They attribute their signs and symptoms to any number of other conditions.

In the vast majority of cases, an estimated 90%, eight types of food are responsible for the allergic reaction. That is important as it helps individuals successfully monitor and control the types of foods they eat. Imagine if every type of food was an allergen suspect. It would make going to a restaurant virtually impossible!

Reactions to allergens vary greatly by individual depending on the sensitivity to the allergen and the amount consumed. Mild symptoms are similar to those of hay fever sufferers: sneezing, watery eyes, and stuffy nose, although food allergies may also cause stomach cramping and diarrhea.

Severe reactions can be dangerous and even life threatening. They include difficulty breathing, swelling of the tongue or throat which may completely cut off access for breathing, dizziness, fainting, and severe vomiting. If you experience any of these reactions, seek medical assistance immediately.

Did You Know?

Epinephrine is a common treatment for severe allergy attacks. If you suffer food allergies, always make sure to carry epinephrine in an auto injector pen for immediate treatment of symptoms. Also, wear an identification bracelet to alert first responders to your condition.

Dairy

Many people believe that milk allergies are the same as lactose intolerance, but the two are different. Milk allergies are physical reactions to the whey or casein found in cow's milk and in products made with that milk. Lactose intolerance on the other hand is the body's inability to successfully breakdown a natural sugar known as lactose.

True milk allergies are not common in adults. Most are likely to suffer from intolerance to lactose. However, an estimated 3% of children have this allergy. Most will outgrow this condition. Some will not. As a matter of fact, children with milk allergies are more likely to develop allergies to nuts, eggs, and soy than those who do not suffer from such an allergy.

Eggs

If you've done any cooking in your life, you know that most recipes call for eggs. They are everywhere and very difficult to avoid. Even foods that you wouldn't normally attribute with eggs contain eggs in some form or another. The list includes Caesar salad dressing, root beer, soups, lollipops, puddings, and cake frostings, just to name a few. And they may be especially difficult to find because they can be labeled under pseudonyms like albumin, globulin, lysozyme, and ovalbumin.

For most people who suffer with egg allergies, they are allergic to the egg whites rather than the yoke. However, all types of egg products should be avoided. Be careful to read all the labels for the food you are eating and avoid anything you're uncertain about.

Fish

Fish allergies are one of the few allergies that commonly develop in adulthood. An estimated 40% of those with the allergy first developed the condition after the age of 18. About half of sufferers have allergies to multiple types of fish.

If you have a fish allergy, it is best to completely avoid all types of fish and refrain from visiting seafood restaurants to avoid the risk of cross contamination.

In most circumstances, it's relatively easy to avoid fish unless you live in a coastal area where that is the main food source. However, there are some surprising places with fish and fish products are lurking. Worcestershire sauce and anything made from it, Caesar salad dressing, and gelatins all contain some type of fish byproduct.

If you have an allergy to fish, understand that you may also have an allergy to shellfish. Don't take a 'try it and find out' approach. Contact a local allergist to get tested to see if you do, indeed, have such an allergy. Knowing in advance can greatly reduce the risk of a severe life threatening allergic reaction.

Peanuts

For patients who suffer from peanut allergies, their bodies mistake the peanut as a harmful substance triggering a protective response from the immune system. Depending on the severity of the response, the results can be life threatening.

The only way to official diagnose a peanut allergy is to see an allergist for evaluation. He will run a series of tests to determine the cause of you reaction.

Once diagnosed, you should avoid produces containing peanuts. Because this is a fairly common allergy many foods are clearly labeled to indicate whether peanuts are present. Many restaurants as well have begun identifying foods made with peanut products.

Shellfish

There are two main types of shellfish, crustaceans and mollusks, each with unique proteins. Crustaceans include lobsters, crabs, shrimp, and crayfish. Squid, oysters, snails, and clams make up the mollusk family. People with an allergy to shellfish may have an allergy unique to one particular food or may be allergic to the entire food group.

Just like with fish allergies, if you suffer from a shellfish allergy, you should stir clear of seafood restaurants, you should also be very cautious about restaurants which serve fish or shellfish on the menu as there could be an instance of cross contamination.

Lastly, keep your distance when shellfish are being prepared. Avoid situations where shellfish are being prepared. Inhaling the steam from cooking can be enough to trigger an allergic reaction in some people.

Soy

Soy allergies are fairly common. These allergies typically manifest in children and infants as a reaction to soy-based infant formulas. For most children, they eventually grow out of the allergy with no lasting effects.

Individuals with a history of allergies are at the greatest risk for developing this type of allergy. Age is another factor. Although it is possible for adults to develop an allergy to soy, it is uncommon. Also, individuals who suffer from other types of allergies are susceptible to soy allergies. This is especially true for individuals with allergies to wheat, legumes, or milk.

Avoid foods with soy or soy products. Read food labels carefully. Some types of bread contain soy four. Crackers and cereals are commonly made with soy flour. Canned soups, low fat peanut butter, processed meats, canned tuna, Worcestershire sauce, and vegetable oils are also common sources for hidden soy products.

Tree Nuts

Allergies to tree nuts can occur in both children and adults and tend to be lifelong issues. Only an estimated 9% of children with this allergy will outgrow it. And research suggests that this type of allergy runs in families. Siblings of tree nut allergy sufferers tend to be at a greater risk for this allergy than those who have no allergic relation.

As the name implies, tree nuts include all nuts which grow on trees. This includes pecans, walnuts, almonds, hazelnuts, cashew, and Brazil nuts. While an individual may only be allergic to a specific nut, it is best to avoid all types of nuts as the allergic reactions can be quite severe.

Carefully read all labels and avoid any product that clearly mentions a nut of any kind. Be mindful that some types of alcoholic beverage contain nut byproducts including nut flavorings. Also, many energy bars and flavored coffees are made from nut flavoring.

Wheat

People who suffer from wheat allergies have a difficult time avoiding wheat entirely. Like with eggs, wheat is practically everywhere. A vast majority of the products we typically eat contain some form of wheat.

Most people would only think about breads and cereals as the primary wheat product we eat on a daily basis. However, wheat can be found in ketchup, cold cuts, soy sauce, beer, ice cream, and even licorice.

Most people who suffer with wheat allergies are able to tolerate oats and rye. They must modify their diets to accommodate the allergy by cooking with either of these two ingredients and avoiding wheat completely.

Wheat allergies are most common in babies and small children who have yet to develop a fully mature immune system. Typically, they will grow out of it although it can manifest itself well into adulthood.

Indoor Household Allergens

In Chapter 4, we discussed some of the toxins that may be lurking and around your home. But did you know that your home might be a haven for allergens. You could unknowingly be contributing to the onset of an allergy attack. Mold, dust mites, and animal dander are all common household allergens that hide even in the cleanest homes.

No home is completely immune to household allergens, but there are steps you can take to mitigate the allergens in your home. (And, no, you won't have to get rid of Fluffy!)

Allergy Proof Your Home

To allergy proof your home start at the floor and work your way up. Remove carpeting which may contain formaldehyde and install quality hardwood flooring. Use area rugs that may be washed regularly. Choose linoleum or tile for the kitchens and bathrooms. If that is not possible, vacuum at least weekly. Families with pets should vacuum at least twice a week or more.

Choose furniture that is easily cleaned. Avoid upholstered furniture and instead choose pieces made from leather, wood, plastic, or metal. Bedding should be washed weekly to remove dust mites. Replace pillows every eight to twelve months. Avoid using strain resisters on furniture as these may contain chemicals that can trigger an allergy attack.

Remove clutter from your home. Clutter attracts dust and dirt. Knickknacks should be put away and stored, if not donated to a local charity. Remove old magazines and books from tables. Avoid keeping a bookcase in your bedroom because books are known mold breading grounds. Keep it in the den or study and vacuum it regularly.

Keep windows closed during allergy season. Run the HVAC instead. Change filters monthly (more often during allergy season) to maximize the quality of air circulating through the home.

If your walls are papered, consider removing the old wallpaper and painting. Wash walls weekly and check for signs of mold or mildew. For small areas, it may be possible to use a bleach or vinegar solution to clean the area and prevent further contamination.

In the basement, check the foundation and walls for signs of leaks. Make repairs immediately. Install a dryer vent that vents air outside. Finally use a dehumidifier to remove the dampness from the air. This will help prevent mold and mildew from forming.

Know Your Triggers

For people with allergies, avoiding allergens is a part of life. Learn what triggers your allergy attacks and how to minimize your exposure. Take proper precautions to avoid food allergens and make sure you always have an epinephrine pen available in case of an accidental exposure.

Make your home an allergy free home. Take steps to reduce the number of allergens you are exposed to throughout your entire home but especially in your bedroom. When possible, avoid perfumes and commercial fragrances as these can often trigger an allergy attack.

A Happy Belly

During my quest for good health, my doctor recommended I take a food allergen test. At the time of the test I was eating lots of fruits and vegetables, so I thought, I'm eating right why would I have any food allergens? Well I'm glad I took the test because I found out I had sensitivity to 23 different foods. And unfortunately, most of my sensitivity was directly at healthy foods like spinach and different types of beans.

That made healing my digestive system a bit more challenging but I was determined. I learned that people who take multiple antibiotics can suffer from more digestive irregularity. The reason for this is that the antibiotics kill the natural bacteria in your gut. As fate would have it, I had taken several antibiotics throughout my lifetime, which was one of the root causes of the food allergens I now faced. Add that to the sensitivity and having to eliminate the health foods I was eating made healing my gut an even bigger challenge.

I experimented with different types of probiotics and found that papaya enzymes are the only ones gentle enough for me. You may benefit from other forms commonly found in yogurts, but those tended to elevate my level of anxiety.

Chapter 8 Common Health Conditions

As we learned in Chapter 2, endocrine disorders play a major role in mood and anxiety disorders. There are numerous health conditions and diseases that directly affect the endocrine system and hormonal balance. These conditions can play havoc with your emotional well-being.

Unfortunately, we don't always realize that we have health problems until signs arise. And all too often we don't actually see the warning signs when they're present. We mistake them for other things or as the simple signs of aging. In this chapter, we'll look at some common health conditions and how they affect the anxiety you feel.

Anemia

Anemia is a condition caused by the body's inability to produce enough healthy red blood cells to function properly. The most common reason for the condition is an insufficient amount of iron; however anemia can also occur from a lack of B12, magnesium, or folic acid. In fact, there are numerous types of vitamin deficiencies that can lead to anemia.

The symptoms of anemia closely mimic those of an anxiety disorder. Symptoms include heart flutters, fatigue, weakness, and shortness of breath. Many people only learn of their anemic condition during treatment for anxiety. And vice versa. Some people have convinced themselves they have anemia rather than facing the realization they have a 'mental disorder.' For those patients, the mere thought of an anxiety disorder causes anxiety.

Anemia is a common condition, affecting up to 10% of the population. It is especially common in pregnant women. Most of those women will fully recover after delivery.

Make no mistake about it, this can be a serious condition. Depending on the type and level deficiency involved, patients may require hospitalization to elevate vitamin levels to a functioning level. This is particularly true if the anemia deficiency was caused by and in conjunction with another serious medical condition such as advanced kidney disease, lupus, diabetes, or hypothyroidism.

For most people, a balanced diet will help correct the anemic condition. However, you should consult a doctor regularly to monitor deficiency levels and rule out any other medical conditions.

Did You Know?

In order to accurately check for anemia, you must test all four iron levels. To do this, you must test ferritin, % saturation, TLBC, and total iron.

Asthma

Asthma is a condition in which breathing is difficult or impossible due to an inflammation of the airways. These attacks may be difficult to manage and may be life threatening if treatment is rendered promptly.

There are many things that can trigger an asthma attack and anxiety is one of them. However, you must understand anxiety does not cause asthma. Asthma and anxiety are two separate medical conditions. If you do not have asthma, an anxiety attack will not cause you to suddenly develop the condition.

The same cannot necessarily be said of the reverse. While an asthma attack will not cause an anxiety disorder, it can cause a sufferer to experience an anxiety like event. You may feel like you're having an anxiety attack when you have an asthma attack.

Asthma is a physiological medical condition that should be treated by a licensed physician. Anxiety, as we have seen, is multifaceted and may have numerous different causes and contributing factors. The two cannot and should not be treated as one in the same.

Diabetes

It is possible, though somewhat unlikely, that patients with diabetes may develop an anxiety disorder. This happens primarily in the beginning of treatment, shortly after the patient learns of their diagnosis. The patient begins to worry excessively of the new diagnosis and the quality of life they will continue to have, the worry prevents sleep, and quickly turns into anxiety. In this way, diabetes can cause anxiety.

Diabetes refers to a group of medical conditions that affect how your body processes glucose. It is primarily a disease of the pancreas (we spoke about the pancreas in Chapter 2!) and the body's interaction with insulin. There are several types of diabetes and pre-diabetes which we'll discuss here. Regardless of the type, it is vitally important that you seek medical assistance for treatment. Diabetes can have many adverse effects on your body, most of which are irreversible. Prompt attention and strictly following medical advice can delay or prevent the onset of those conditions.

Type 1

Type 1 diabetes is caused by the body's immune system attacking the pancreatic cells that produce insulin. It is not caused by diet, although people with Type 1 diabetes must carefully monitor their diet for life.

In a perfectly healthy patient, the glucose from a meal would alert the pancreas to release insulin in proportion to the size of the meal. The insulin would then prepare the sugar to be used in the body's cell. As the glucose is absorbed into the cells throughout the body, the blood sugar levels drop.

This process doesn't even begin in individuals with Type 1 diabetes. Their bodies have already begun attacking the insulin producers in the pancreas so there is no insulin to secrete. Without that insulin, blood sugar levels spike causing a strain on all other parts of the body.

Type 1diabetes may cause dehydration especially when blood sugar levels are at their highest, unexplained weight loss, or damage to the eyes, kidneys, and heart. It has also been known to cause heart attacks and strokes

Most patients with Type 1 diabetes develop the condition early in life, before age 20. Fortunately, it is not a common form of diabetes. Only about 5% of patients diagnosed with diabetes have Type 1. It's more common in Caucasians than in minorities and is equally divided between men and women.

Type 2

Type 2 diabetes is by far the most common form of diabetes diagnosed. Approximately 95% of those who suffer from the disease have Type 2. It affects roughly 26 million Americans. Some people may know it by its former common name, non-insulin-dependent diabetes.

Unlike Type 1, this form of diabetes does not involve the immune system. It may be caused by a number of factors that either prevent the pancreas from making enough insulin or prevent the body from fully utilizing the insulin. This causes a spike in blood sugar levels which can cause additional damage throughout the body.

Damage to the pancreas is a main factor in the development of Type 2 diabetes. Damage may be caused by any number of factors including illness or injury but is more often the result of poor diet. Individuals who routinely eat diets high in processed sugars and carbohydrates often tax the pancreas repeatedly. Over time, this will cause damage to the insulin producing cells.

If left untreated, Type 2 diabetes can cause any number of health complications including diabetic coma, damage to the kidneys, eyes, and heart, or hardening the arteries. Like Type 1, Type 2 diabetes is a complex medical condition that requires treatment from your doctor. While diet may play a major role in treatment, you should not attempt to self-treat this condition with dietary changes.

Hyperglycemia

Hyperglycemia occurs when blood sugar levels reach or exceed 200 mg/dL. This can develop into a dangerous condition if levels remain this high for a prolonged period of time.

Early symptoms include frequent urination, headaches, fatigue, and blurred vision. Symptoms from prolonged elevated levels include nausea, vomiting, weakness, confusion, abdominal pain, and eventually coma.

There may be any number of causes for hyperglycemia. Some patients experience the condition after surgery or injury. It is a common side effect from steroids. It may be due to a poor diet or an inadequate level of exercise. Or, it may be brought on by emotional stress.

Excessively high blood sugar levels can jeopardize overall health. If you experience any of these signs or symptoms, it is a good idea to consult with a physician who can thoroughly evaluate blood sugar levels and overall health.

Hypoglycemia

Unlike other forms of diabetic disorders, hypoglycemia is the result of low blood sugar instead of an elevated blood sugar level. There are several known causes of hypoglycemia including diet, excessive exercise, and certain medications.

Individuals who suffer from hypoglycemia suffer a wide range of symptoms that they may not recognize as a serious medical condition. They generally experience confusion or fuzziness when completing routine tasks, dizziness, uncontrollable hunger, headaches, weakness, and anxiety. Without proper treatment, hypoglycemia can develop more serious symptoms including poor coordination, blackouts, and even coma.

Certain diabetic drugs have been known to cause a hypoglycemia episode. Patients whose medication causes a drastic drop in blood sugar are likely to experience hypoglycemic symptoms. These medications include chlorpropamide, tolbutamide, warfarin, and allopurinol.

Another form of hypoglycemia is reactive hypoglycemia, a condition in which blood sugar levels drop significantly in non diabetic patients after they eat a meal. This drop in blood sugar may occur while fasting or after each meal. In many cases, it is not a permanent condition and can be corrected by improving one's diet. Symptoms are similar to diabetic hypoglycemia. They include weakness, hunger, sleepiness, confusion, anxiety, and lightheadedness. For some individuals, the supplement chromium picolinate in doses of 200-300mg taken with each meal works well to help prevent blood sugar drops.

Insomnia

Insomnia can be considered the Yin/Yang to anxiety. It can cause anxiety as well as be caused by anxiety. It creates a perfect circle and sometimes it may be difficult to determine which condition came first.

For insomniacs, the condition feels uncontrollable. They want to sleep. In fact, they're usually desperate for sleep, but they can't seem to sleep once they crawl into bed.

Prescription medications and supplements such as melatonin may offer relief. That being said, a better strategy for dealing with insomnia is to take control of the situation and make some permanent lifestyle changes.

Go running before you sit down for dinner or earlier in the day. As we learned in Chapter 5, exercise releases endorphins which create a natural high. It also gives your body a reason to shut down. It's tired and wants to rest.

Try eating lighter meals at night. This will give your digestive system plenty of time to process the large meal you eat throughout the day. Also, not having a heavy meal on your stomach will prevent indigestion and heartburn from keeping you awake. Limit the amount of liquids you drink three to four hours prior to bedtime.

Create a regular bed time and set it in stone. Remember as a kid when your mother made you go to bed at 9p.m.? She was right! A regular bedtime helps reset your body's internal clock. Your body will not want to stay up because it's used to resting during that time. If you find that you can't fall asleep after thirty minutes, get up and read a non excitable book with a dim reading light. Once you start to feel drowsy, go back to bed. Keep this cycle up until you fall asleep.

Limit your TV intake at night. About one hour prior to bedtime, turn off the television and all other electronic devises. Read a book or magazine that is not related to work and will not cause you to be overly stimulated. Or try lying on a heating pad with all the lights in the room off while you meditate.

Lastly, keep a 'blessings journal' by your bed. Many people find it difficult to turn their minds off at night. They tend to focus on all the problems of the day and the challenges ahead. Keep a journal by your bed each night and list five things you are thankful for. It can be anything that you consider a blessing in your life. This simple exercise will help you refocus on the positive aspects of your life and go to bed with positive thoughts instead of negative ones.

> **Did You Know?**
>
> **Large amounts of melatonin can disrupt your sleep. Using as little as 1mg helps to mimic your body's natural melatonin production.**

Lupus

Many people who have lupus also develop an anxiety condition although the two conditions are not directly connected. One does not cause the other. Not all individuals who suffer from Lupus have anxiety although many of them do develop the condition as a result of stress from the disease.

Lupus is an autoimmune disease in which the body begins to attack itself. The typical patient is female during the age of reproduction. It's an unpredictable disease in that it can flare up at any time. Lupus is a chronic disease which makes exercise and physical fitness difficult at best. It is this sedentary lifestyle which may add to the depression and anxiety of sufferers.

Additionally, lupus causes anxiety like symptoms to arise from out of the blue. Patients may experience difficulty breathing, fogginess, and chest pains which mimic the symptoms of an anxiety attack.

Lastly many of the medicines commonly used to treat lupus cause anxiety. It is one of the primary side effects of treatment. In this case, it could be that the medicine is the direct link between lupus and anxiety and not the disease itself. One of the few drugs which does not cause anxiety is Low Dose Naltrexone. It is a wonder drug for auto-immune disease, especially if taken in doses of 1.5 - 4.5mg.

Menopause

In Chapter 2, we learned about the complexities of the hormonal network in women. Women face a plethora of mental issues brought on by our hormones throughout our lives. That is particularly true during menopause. It is a time when our bodies go through a drastic hormonal fluctuation.

Women in menopause often experience anxiety as a direct result to the changes they are undergoing. Along with hot flashes, anxiety seems to be a fairly common experience. The good news is after menopause, anxiety seems to disappear unless the woman suffered from the condition prior to menopause. Even then, in some case, the anxiety disappears completely.

Many women find that coping with the anxiety as it occurs is an effective treatment. Others chose to incorporate exercise into their normal routine. There are numerous treatments that work effectively for combating the symptoms of anxiety induced by menopause.

MTHFR Gene Mutation

If you're like most people, you've never heard of MTHFR gene mutation. It stands for methylenetetrahydrofolate reductase gene. (Thank goodness it's abbreviated!!) There are actually two MTHFR's in the human body, one is a gene, and the other is an enzyme.

So what does the MTHFR gene do? Its primary function is to unlock the MTHFR enzyme. When this doesn't happen properly, serious symptoms can arise. Conditions such as asthma, center types of cancers, heart murmurs and heart attacks, Alzheimer's migraines, and Type 1 diabetes just to name a few.

Many doctors have little working knowledge of this condition despite its seriousness. If you are concerned about MTHFR gene mutation and believe it could be the cause of any of your medical conditions, contact the medical associations in your area to find a doctor with experience in the field.

Science or Dogma?

We've learned quite a bit on our journey for the root cause of anxiety. One question that comes to my mind, especially after all we've learned thus far, "Are the principles of modern American medicine guided by science or dogma?"

Let me explain what I mean by that question.

Science is a system of thoughts in which observers collect data, test that data for reproducibility, and construct theories using the simplest explanation to explain the results. Anyone can make a new observation that leads to a breakthrough in any scientific field.

In the medical profession, the greatest discoveries

are often made in the offices of regular doctors practicing their chosen craft. These are the people who are actively working with patients. They see real patients with real symptoms. While each physician has a different level of knowledge and experience in certain areas, they all understand the differences between medical theory and clinical medicine. They experience that on a daily basis.

Dogma is something different. It relies on the information we know today to rigidly define the truths of tomorrow. It fails to account for observations that are inconsistent with its line of belief. Its truths are absolute.

I'm concerned that the medical profession has become dogmatic. Today medicine is taught as an absolute and not an ever evolving quest for knowledge. There is a general disregard within the profession for anything that is not fully understood. Such observations must be false because they have yet to be proven. The proof lies in the way modern medicine and alternative medicine interact and compete against one another. They two should not be on competitive sides of a dogmatic argument. They should work together to improve the quality of life for the patients they serve.

Chapter 9 Tracking the Root Cause

We've covered quite a bit of information on our journey together. We now know the different hormones and neurotransmitters that affect you mood. We can recognize toxins and allergens that are lurking in your home and take steps to limit your exposure. We understand how exercise and the foods you eat can influence how you feel throughout the entire day. And we know what health conditions can cause an anxiety disorder or an anxiety attack.

Now, we need to determine which of these conditions apply to you so that you can take active steps to combat your anxiety issues. I have divided the tests into two distinct sections, Required Tests and Suggested Tests. Recognizing that some of these tests are rather expensive if you do not have medical insurance and may not be covered by all insurance plans, I would encourage following through with the suggested tests only if your particular situation warrants the expense.

The first course of action you should take is to see your doctor for a complete physical. Strongly request tests that will rule out the health conditions we discussed in Chapter 8, especially a fasting and non-fasting blood sugar test to rule out diabetes. Once you eliminate common diseases and health conditions, you can begin to eliminate the other issues we have discussed.

One last thing I'd like to mention, keep a temperature log. People with thyroid disorders tend to run slightly higher or lower temperatures than average. Therefore, it is recommended that you maintain a body temperature log for at least a week prior to your doctor's visit. Measure your temperature each morning before you get out of bed. Body temperatures tend to change throughout the day with activity and external environmental conditions but in the morning your body will display the most accurate temperature without the interference from these factors. A glass thermometer is most accurate. It's recommended to log your temperature every three hours throughout the day, beginning when you first wake up and then consistently throughout the day. If your average daily temperature is less than the normal of 98.6 degrees, then you more than likely have a thyroid condition. Be sure to check your temperatures at least 30 minutes before or after a meal and at least 15 minutes before or after drinking anything.

Required Tests

The tests in this section are essential to uncovering issues regarding your entire endocrine system.

Adrenal Cortisol Test

To accurately test your cortisol levels use a saliva test four times a day. These can be purchased online at a relatively inexpensive rate. Saliva tests taken throughout the day create a more accurate portrait of your actual cortisol levels. Remember, in Chapter 2 we discussed how these levels fluctuate throughout the day. Just remember, to receive an accurate reading you will need to stop all cortisol containing supplements for at least seven days prior to the test. If you are on cortisol containing medication, you will need to work closely with your doctor to slowly wean off the medication prior to the test.

Test Your T's

As we discussed in Chapter 2, your thyroid gland produces two main hormones which greatly impact mood and anxiety, thyroxine and triiodothyronine. It is vital therefore to check these levels especially if you have any of the signs and symptoms mentioned earlier. For the most accurate results you should take these tests at the same time.

Free T3

To measure the level of triiodothyronine in your system you will need to have a free T3 conducted. Check with your physician as this may be a standard test that has been taken during your physical.

Reverse T3

This test is used to measure the inactive form of T3 to determine the exact efficiency of your thyroid. In many states this can be taken without a doctor's order. This test is a must have with all thyroid panels you take.

A high reading on your reverse T3 test may be indicative of Hashimoto's Thyroiditis or hypothyroidism. It may also indicate problems with the adrenal glands. If your levels are high, make sure you also test your cortisol levels as well as your T4. Many doctors will only address the reverse T3 issue and will not look further to find the underlying cause.

Free T4

The other major hormone produced by the thyroid is thyroxine. Your free T4 panel will check those levels.

TSH

This test is used to determine if you suffer from hypopituitarism. It measures the level of TSH to ensure there is not a hidden culprit for a thyroid irregularity. TSH alone does not accurately test for thyroid disfunction.

Thyroid Antibodies

You should also test the thyroid antibodies to rule out Hashimoto's disease. In order to do that you will need to take the Anti-TPO and TgAb tests. For added peace of mind, also take a TSI series at the same time rule out Grave's disease.

Did You Know?

Many undiagnosed thyroid patients, or those patients taking the thyroid replacement hormones, still report not feeling quite 'right'. They just don't feel well. For many people, merely being in the 'normal' range is not enough. They are not at their optimal levels.

So, what levels are considered 'optimal' by most Functional Medicine physicians?

Free T3 – Within the top 25th percentile range
Reverse T3 – Low end of normal
Free T4 – Top ½ of the referenced range
TSH- Less than 2.0
Thyroid Peroxidase Antibodies (TPO) – Within the referenced range
Vitamin D –Over 50
Ferritin – Over 60 (With hair loss, over 80)

Iron

You should also check the level's of iron in your system to determine whether your body is absorbing the necessary amount. Avoid iron supplements for at least five days prior to testing to ensure an accurate reading. To accurately test the iron levels, run an iron series including Ferritin, Saturation %, TIBC, and Serum Iron. If your Ferritin is less than 50, your levels are too low.

Vitamins

As we've learned earlier, your body needs certain vitamins and minerals to function properly and produce the necessary hormones and neurotransmitters. Make sure you test your vitamin D3 levels by running a 25-Hydroxy Vitamin D and a Vitamin D3 di-OH. And most importantly, Calcitriol (25 di-OH Vitamin D) which tests for the active form of D. Additionally, you will need to test if your vitamin B12 is working correctly by having a Folate test.

Suggested Tests

Depending on the results of your previous tests, you may require additional testing to fully determine the root cause for your anxiety issues. These tests will greatly assist you in your quest. In addition to the tests mentioned here, both men and women should have their reproductive hormones tested to ensure they are in normal ranges for their age.

Electrolytes

Run a complete electrolyte series to ensure that your essential vitamins are in line with normal levels. Tests should include RBC Magnesium, RBC Potassium, Calcium, Sodium, and Glucose. As we're learned throughout the book, your body cannot function without these vital elements. If any of them are out of balance, your entire system will be out of balance.

Parathyroid

If your calcium levels are high or you suspect this issue, check your parathyroid as well to see if that is the root cause of the imbalance.

MTHFR Gene

This test is particularly important if your tests showed a high reading of mercury, copper, lead, iron, or B12. Furthermore, if you have a family history of cancer, heart disease, or autoimmune conditions, this test may help you uncover a serious underlying problem.

Author's Note:

Two of my personal favorite books on this topic are *Stop the Thyroid Madness* by Janie Alexander Bowthorpe and *Recovering with T3* by Paul Robinson. Both books work to dispel the medical myths surrounding the thyroid and thyroid medications. I regularly recommend both books to clients and know that you will gain a wealth of knowledge should you choose to explore these works further.

Chapter 10 Natural Treatment Options

Finding the root cause of your anxiety is only half the battle. Once you know what to address, you can begin making positive lifestyle changes to improve your overall quality of life. With some fairly simple steps you will be amazed at how effectively you can overcome much of your anxiety without the use of anti-anxiety medication.

You should understand that no life, no matter how perfect, is completely stress free. There will be times when stress plays a major factor in your life. You may experience a family illness, your job may require extra hours, or you may have relationship difficulties. Whatever the stressors are, you should understand that these are normal. Everyone experiences stress on some level. Learning to recognize and manage the stress before it becomes a major problem is the essential key in leading a healthy and productive life. Once you have addressed the root causes of your condition and incorporated the following lifestyle changes, you will be prepared to meet the demands of your life without succumbing to anxiety again.

Also understand that not all techniques will work for everyone. You may respond well to diet and exercise while another person may see more success with mediation and mental anxiety exercises. That's okay. There's no one-size-fits-all in anxiety relief. Try these techniques in conjunction with addressing the root causes of your particular anxiety problem. Once you find the combination that works well for you, you'll be amazed at how much better your life will become.

Combat the Problem Head On

The first and most effective step in overcoming anxiety is to tackle the problem directly. Admittedly, this approach may seem somewhat counterintuitive and definitely well outside your comfort zone. The last thing you want to do when you're in the midst of a full fledged panic attack is to directly address the demon itself.

And that's why this technique works so well because the demon within your anxiety attack doesn't want you to address it directly. It feeds off its ability to fight in the shadows of your psyche. Therefore, when you combat it head on, you take away its power and control over you.

Learn to recognize the initial signs of a panic attack. When you feel the first symptoms, focus on your breathing. Deeply inhale and slowly exhale counting each breath during the process. Complete at least ten deep breaths to calm and relax your body.

Once your body is relaxed, focus on the negative thoughts that are bombarding your mind. Chances are, the stereo in your mind is blasting a constant stream of harsh criticisms. Change the channel. Envision yourself physically changing the channel on the stereo. The new station plays a repetitive mantra. It may be, "I can do this" or "I am not going to fail." It may be your favorite Bible verse or inspirational quote. Whatever touches and inspires you to do well. Repeat it over and over again until the attack has passed.

It may take several attempts before this technique is fully effective. Panic attacks can be scary. It's difficult to overcome that fear initially, but with practice and when combined with the other techniques mentioned here, you will be able to combat your panic attacks head on.

Create a Mantra

As we mentioned in the previous section, you will need a mantra to address the negativity and fear you face. This is not only a saying that you will use during a panic attack; it is something you will tell yourself during much of the day even when things are going well. It may be embroidered on a hanging in your kitchen or stenciled in your bathroom so that you'll see it every day. It will become a part of who you are.

Stay Positive

Focus on the positives in your life. This is not the time to give any energy to negativity. For example, it's better to say, "I'm calm and collected" than to say "I won't have another panic attack." The former focuses on what you want to be and will become while the latter reaffirms the fear you feel. Do not give credence to your fears.

Keep It Real

A mantra will do no good if you don't use it. Therefore, keep it real and useable. It should be applicable to your life. If you decide to take up running, you might try telling yourself, "I'm the fastest person on the track." That's great until someone who's run for years beats you without even breaking a sweat. Instead, create a mantra that you can use regardless of the challenges you face. "I am developing a strong, lean body." Remember, you're not competing with anyone nor are you trying to impress anyone with your mantra. You are trying to focus on bettering yourself.

Patience and Dedication

Finally, once you have created a mantra that works for you, use it consistently. When you wake up in the morning, mentally repeat your mantra before you get out of bed. Have it strategically placed throughout you home and office so you see it during the day. Use it as a screen saver on your computer. Repeat it before you go to bed. The more you fill your mind with positive thoughts, the less room there will be for negative thoughts. It's not just a phrase to use during a panic attack; it's a new way to visualize yourself and your future.

Meditate

Regular mediation is one of the most effective methods for alleviating long term anxiety symptoms without medication. Unfortunately, it's also the most misunderstood method. Far too many people envision new age gurus sitting cross-legged repeating chants. While there are those who practice that technique routinely, mediation does not have to involve such complexities. It is a simple practice of clearing your mind of all distractions and focusing on your body.

The easiest form of mediation to begin with is a simple breathing mediation technique. Sit comfortably in a quiet place. Most people will choose a straight backed chair. Do not slouch or slump. You want to keep you body elongated and centered.

Set a timer for a reasonable amount of time, say five minutes to begin with, and increase the time as you become more comfortable with the mediation. Close your eyes and breathe naturally, in through your nose and out through your mouth. You're not trying to control your breathing. You are only going to focus on it.

Focus on how the air travels through your nose, down your trachea, and finally into your lungs. How does it feel as it leaves your body? Repeat the process for each breath. Clear your mind of all other thoughts except the breath entering and leaving your body. It may seem very strange at first because our minds are naturally so busy with day to day tasks that we don't take time to focus on anything in particular but with regular practice, you will be able to clear your mind of all other thoughts. As you improve, you may find that other mediation techniques increase the calmness in your mind. There are many techniques which use progressive muscle relaxation and audio therapy to increase the success of the mediation process. Many people also find that Yoga and Tai Chi are excellent meditative exercises that help center the mind and body.

The most important thing about incorporating mediation into your lifestyle is consistency. Set aside time (even if it's only five minutes!) each day to mediate and focus on calming your mind and body. Calming your mind daily will help prevent future anxiety attacks from occurring.

Don't Forget Your Support Group

Alone time can be a great way to recharge your batteries. Too much alone time on the other hand, can give you too many opportunities to dwell on the negative aspects of your life. If you begin to feel yourself slipping back into your darker moods, reconnect with your friends and social group. Go out to a movie or have dinner with a friend. We are social creatures by natures. It's the way each of us was designed. We all need social interaction to feel connected and emotionally healthy.

If you haven't established a strong social group in your current location, consider some other options to get back out there. Volunteer at a local charity. They would be glad for the assistance and you will get a natural 'helper's high' from the experience. (Those happy hormones kicking in again!)

Try reconnecting with lost family members. Do you have some cousins you haven't seen in years? Try visiting each other and catching up on old times. The same is true for long lost friends. Find your old college roommate and get together for lunch. Or you could look for clubs in your areas of interest that meet locally. Almost every city has some type of social and recreational center where organizations can get together. Maybe you've always wanted to get into coin collecting. There may be an organization in your town that could give you expert advice. Do you enjoy reading? Your library may have information on a local book club.

Lastly, get involved in your local church or synagogue. Research has found that individuals who were active in their religious organization reported far less depression and anxiety than those who weren't. Some studies suggest the reduction could be as much as half. People who actively practice a religion report feeling more connected with their community and more secure in their own lives.

Author's Note:

I am a devoted follower of Jesus Christ and am an active member at my church and have been for many years. This was not always the case. Although I developed a strong faith at an early age, I made choices and mistakes along the way. I don't live in regret over the choices I've made, I have repented and I know Jesus has forgiven me and it's because of Him that I turned my life around. In 2010 I heard the Lord speak so clearly in my ear and he said "Michele I want you off those meds." I knew he meant the benzo and I knew it was what I needed to do. It took a year and a half to finally get up the courage to seek treatment to do it, but I did and it was one of the best decisions I've ever made. And of course it was because it was what God wanted me to do and God is always faithful and always just.

I can personally attest that it was my faith which got me through many difficult times both during my youth and in my dealing with anxiety and benzodiazepine dependency. I could have NEVER of worked a full-time management job, volunteered with children's church on a weekly basis, and been the mother and wife I have been for my family, all while detoxing off a benzo and then anti-depressant if it wasn't for the Lord's strength and guidance. I am humbled by this experience and I now know why I went through all this and it was to help YOU.

Sweat Away Anxiety

As we learned in Chapter 5, exercise if the body's way to chemically fight off anxiety and depression. Physical exercise increases the production and release of endorphins in the brain. These endorphins naturally enhance mood and relieve anxiety and depression.

Remember, start out slowly especially if you've been inactive for many years. Try going on a 15 to 20 minute walk to begin with. Then increase your time as your body adapts to the new exercise. Once you're comfortable with one exercise, you can add new programs and vary your routine. You will begin to reap the benefits of becoming more physically fit, but exercising in this case is not only about physical fitness. It is an opportunity for you to clear your mind and stimulate positive hormonal balance. Don't forget that walking at a moderate pace for 20 minutes a day has been shown to have the same anti-anxiety benefits as a .25mg Xanax! Sweat your way to peace of mind.

Eat a Healthy Diet

It is impossible to reiterate enough how important a healthy and balanced diet is to maintain a healthy body. We learned a great deal about diet in Chapter 5, but you have to put those things into practice if you want to see the results you desire. Also, make sure you start phasing out or reducing any of the foods your body may be dependent on. As we learned in Chapter 6, these foods provide little, if any, nutritional value but greatly inhibit your body's natural rhythm.

Remember to include foods in your diet such as fish, nuts, and spinach which have all been shown to increase mood and decrease depression and anxiety. If you don't like or can't eat a particular food or food group, look for alternative foods which provide similar nutrients. Your body will thank you for it.

And don't forget what Hippocrates said all those years ago, "Let thy food by thy medicine and they medicine be thy food."

Get Plenty of Sleep

We learned in Chapter 2 that hormonal balance and sleep go hand in hand. You can't have one without the other. Therefore, it is essential to get plenty of rest each night. On average, the typical adult should get seven to eight hours of sleep each night. Obviously, there will be times when you're schedule is in disarray or you are under the weather and may get more of less, but on an average day, you should try to get seven to eight hours of sleep.

If you have trouble getting enough sleep on a nightly basis, try to unwind at least two hours before you go to bed. Turn off your computer. Unplug your electronic devices. Don't answer your cell phone. Create a relaxing, sleep inducing environment within your home.

Avoid caffeine late in the day. If you're a soda and coffee drinker, consider switching to caffeine free sodas and teas for your afternoon beverages. Caffeine has no flavor so the taste is exactly the same, but avoiding caffeine after 2p.m. can greatly improve your ability to sleep.

Also, stay away from the alcohol within two hours of bedtime. Some experts say an alcoholic beverage is fine with dinner or with friends, but going to sleep immediately after alcohol consumption will disrupt your sleep patterns. You may fall asleep faster, but the sleep will be more fitful and result in waking up during the middle of the night.

> **Author's Note:**
>
> **If you suffer from anxiety, I highly recommend giving up all caffeine and alcoholic beverages. I have and it's made a tremendous difference in the levels of anxiety I feel!**

Organize

Your home is your castle, your protective buffer for the stressors of the world outside and your shelter for family and friends. It should be a peaceful place, a place you want to come home to and invite people into. Unfortunately, clutter and disorder can diminish that peaceful harmony.

Clutter in your home or office can greatly increase the level of anxiety you feel on a daily basis. This is true whether you consider yourself a neat freak or you prefer your home to have a lived-in feel. Scientists who have studied clutter and hoarding have found links in the amount of clutter a person has in their home with the level of anxiety and depression they feel. Clutter raises stress hormones (remember what we learned in Chapter 2!) and increases blood pressure.

Not sure how to start to organize your home? Start simply. Just like deciding to lose weight, decluttering takes a bit of time. Begin by incorporating a new habit into your daily routine. For example, vow to make your bed every morning or to wash the dishes immediately after a meal to avoid leaving them in the sink. Each day, regardless of how tired you are or how you'd like to catch an extra ten minutes of shuteye, complete the task for your new habit. Do this for a week, then on the first day of the second week, add another task to it. It could be something as simple as wiping off the counters in your bathroom each morning or night. It could be sweeping the kitchen floor daily. Continue to practice the habit you began in the first week, but incorporate a new habit weekly until you have a pattern of cleanly habits that you do daily or every other day, depending on the activity.

Next, you'll need to tackle some bigger projects such as getting rid of some excess stuff. Once a week, choose a project to complete. Perhaps, you need to you have a project you've wanted to tackle like cleaning out the refrigerator or pantry. Maybe you want to take some of your old clothes to a local charity. Pick one project that you can complete within a few hours and do it.

By merely opening up the space in your home, you will begin to feel a weight lifting off your chest. And best of all, with less clutter, your home will be less susceptible to indoor allergens and toxins which may be adding to your physical and emotional discomfort. Organization is a win-win situation for defeating anxiety!

Forget the Joneses!!

Too many people focus on the happiness of others and begin to feel inferior because their lives don't seem to measure up. Social media only adds fuel to that fire. Each day, through your Twitter feed, Instagram, and Facebook posts, you can see who got the latest sports car, who had an amazing birthday bash, or who just got a promotion at work. It's enough to leave anyone feeling a bit blah about the day-to-day humdrum activities of a wife and mother. Or the father stuck in a dead end job he hates for that matter.

Remember, life is not a contest to see who can gain the most possessions. As a matter of fact, I just told you to get rid of that excess stuff! Life is a journey to discover emotional balance and well-being. You can't be harmonious if you're always trying to get the latest gadget to impress someone else.

As of this moment, STOP IT!

Repeat after me, "My life is more important that material possessions."

Each time you see the latest and greatest gizmo, repeat that phrase. Write it on a slip of paper to put it next to your credit cards in your purse or wallet. Then, the next time you feel the impending urge to buy something that's sure to impress everyone around you, read that statement five times.

Another way to combat the Jones syndrome is to limit your time on social media. This is especially true if social media causes you to feel anxious or depressed as the wonderful lives of others. Instead of catching up with friends online, go out and catch up with them in real life. Face time with friends is a great way to relieve stress and keep you grounded about what really matters.

Set Goals for Yourself

All too often, we get caught up in the 'what ifs' and the potential for negative outcomes in our daily lives. One positive method to counteract those negative thoughts is by setting realistic goals for yourself. Research has shown that goal setting and completing tasks gives us a great sense of accomplishment which triggers the production of happy hormones in the brain.

It is important to note that the goals must be realistic! You can't simply set the goal of winning the lottery or dating a famous celebrity as your main goal and expect to check those items off your list. Sure they may be fun, but the likelihood of either of those coming to fruition is rather slim to put it mildly.

Set goals that are important to you and will have a positive impact when completed. For example, if your goal is to lose weight and your ultimate goal is to lose 40 pounds, you may have a monthly weight loss goal of five pounds. These are realistic short-term and long-term goals as they are both very accomplishable. Likewise, if your goal is to clean out the garage but it's piled floor to ceiling with long lost treasures, make your short term goal to clean and discard five boxes a week until the project is complete.

Remember, manageable steps are the key to successfully completing any goal. As long as you know you are continuing to move forward and can see the progress of your efforts you will be more likely to keep your anxious feelings at bay.

Supplements

Supplements can be a good way to provide your body with vitamins and nutrients you may not get from your regular diet. This is particularly true if you have a food allergy or sensitivity to certain types of food like dairy products.

It is important to understand, however, that not all supplements are created equally. Currently there are no federal regulations mandating the manufacture of dietary supplements. As such, you must be cautious.

Avoid generic brands if possible. They have routinely been shown to contain additional fillers like sugars which your body doesn't need and can aggravate medical condition like diabetes. Stick with reputable companies and research before you buy. Consumer Reports and Good Housekeeping have both done comparisons on supplements. They can provide a good source of information for the particular supplement you're looking for.

Beating Anxiety for Good!

Ridding your mind and body of anxiety is a never ending battle. There will be times when you still feel stressed and anxious. Life will throw you curveballs and ruin your best laid plans. But you can live a happy and productive life.

Remember, as with all things, this is a journey. Don't give up if it takes you longer to reach your destination than those around you. You are on your own path. Travel it well!

My Supplements

Some of my clients have asked what types of supplements I take considering the different types of health complications I have. Here's a list of the supplements that I take and which have helped me. You may not need these supplements as they may not be right for your health conditions. For the best results, contact a holistic physician who can help outline a specific plan for your unique needs.

Magnesium citrate	Vitamin A, C, & E	Zinc picolinate	Papaya Enzymes
Protandim	Vitamin B1	Chromium picolinate	

At the time of this writing, my medications include Cytomel and Natural Thyroid. Additionally, I needed to get my central nervous system back in check. My doctor prescribed Low Dose Naltrexone (LDN). I was extremely skeptical! After all, my body had just fought and won a major battle caused by the medication I had taken for years, but; it turned out to be extremely beneficial for me.

Naltrexone was originally designed to help drug addicts fight the pains of withdrawal. It was touted as the wonder drug in that field but never fully reached the profit levels the pharmaceutical companies expected. When a drug isn't profitable, the major pharmaceutical companies move on to bigger and brighter stars. But doctors soon realized that the drug had numerous positive effects particularly with autoimmune disorders and issues dealing with the central nervous system. When given in smaller dosages, LDN has helped patients battling cancer, ALS, multiple sclerosis, Parkinson's Disease, Crohn's Disease, and a host of other conditions too plentiful to name here.

I can personally attest to the benefits of this drug. It has helped me immeasurably. And it may be a great treatment option for you if you are experiencing similar symptoms.

Index

Adderall	99
Addison's Disease	36
Adrenal Failure	36-37
Adrenal Fatigue	36
Adrenal Glands	35-39, 42, 102, 133
Alcohol	60, 86-89, 97, 113, 146
Alcohol Abuse	87
Alcoholism	38, 87-88
Allergens	107-109, 114, 116, 131, 147
Almonds	75, 94, 113
Anemia	28, 119-120
Asthma	80, 120-121, 129
Beef	76-77
Benzene	58, 61,
Benzodiazepines	12, 14, 39, 44, 55, 84-85, 100-101, 103-105, 143
Blueberries	77-78, 87
BPA	59-60
Caffeine	36, 89-90, 145-146
Chocolate	78-79
Cortisol	27-28, 35-37, 41-42, 44-46, 48, 78, 132-133
Diabetes	29-30, 32, 42, 75, 93, 120-123, 129, 131, 150,
Diet	21, 26, 34, 36, 41, 47, 50, 52, 59, 61, 71, 74, 77, 79, 80-83, 90-91, 93-95, 114, 120, 122-125, 137, 144-145, 150
Dopamine	49-50, 95, 99, 102

Endocrine System	18-20, 24, 27, 33, 35, 42-43, 51, 54, 59, 119, 132
Endorphins	50-51, 71-72, 126, 144
Epinephrine (Adrenaline)	35, 48, 109, 116
Estrogen	32-33, 38-39, 53, 59
Exercise	10, 34, 36, 51, 58, 71-74, 81, 84, 124, 126-128, 131, 137, 141, 144
Fish (Shellfish)	61-64, 76, 79-80, 110-112, 145
GABA	44, 47, 53-55
Goiters	21-22
Hypopituitarism	27-28, 133
Hyperglycemia	29, 123-124
Hyperparathyroidism	25-26, 28
Hyperthyroidism	22-23
Hypoglycemia	29, 37, 124-125
Hypoparathyroidism	26
Hypothyroidism	23-24, 35, 120, 133
Insomnia	24, 41-42, 45, 65, 89, 100, 125
Iron	76, 119-120, 135-136
Lupus	120, 127-128
Melatonin	35, 40-41, 48, 81, 125, 127
Menopause	128
Mercury	61-70, 79-80, 136
MTHFR Gene Mutation	128-129, 136
Neurotransmitters	47-51, 53-55, 59, 74, 78, 86, 95-97, 100, 131, 135
Norepinephrine	35, 49, 53
Ovaries	19, 27, 32-33, 38-39
Pancreas	19, 29-30, 86, 121-123

Parathyroid	24-26, 30, 75, 136
Peanuts	111
Pineal Gland	35, 40
Pituitary Gland	21, 24, 27-28, 31, 33-34, 37, 40, 42, 50
Progesterone	18, 32-33, 38-39, 43-46, 53-55, 84
Ritalin	13, 99
Serotonin	50-53, 74, 79, 81, 92, 95
Soy	80, 97, 110, 112-114
Sugar	45, 74, 78, 80, 89, 91-95, 110, 122-125, 130, 150
Testes (Testicles)	19, 27, 31-32, 39-40
Testosterone	18, 31, 39-40, 43
Thyroid	18-24, 27, 43, 45, 83-84, 131-134, 136, 151
Wheat	94, 112-114

Find the root cause of your anxiety

Resources & References

Amen, Daniel; *Change Your Brain, Change Your Life: The Breakthrough Program for Conquering Anxiety, Depression, Obsessiveness, Anger, and Impulsiveness;* Harmony; 1999

Bates, Deborah; *Your Personal Tuning Fork: The Endocrine System;* John Hunt Publishing; 2012

Bieling, Peter J. PhD and Ross, Gary S. MD; *Depression and Your Thyroid: What You Need to Know;* New Harbinger Publication, 2006

Cutler, Andrew Hall; *Amalgam Illness, Diagnosis and Treatment : What You Can Do to Get Better, How Your Doctor Can Help;* Andrew Hall Cutler; 1999

Driscoll, Jeanne Watson and Sichel, Deborah; *Women's Moods: What Every Woman Must Know About Hormones, the Brain, and Emotional Health;* Harper Paperbacks; 2000

Drufene, Troy and Watson, Kelly G. PhD; *Things Might Go Terribly, Horribly Wrong: A Guide to Life Liberated from Anxiety;* New Harbinger Publications; 2010

Foldvary-Schaefer, Nancy; *The Cleveland Clinic Guide to Sleep Disorders;* Kaplan Publishing; 2009

Johnsgard, Keith; *Conquering Depression and Anxiety Through Exercise;* Prometheus Books; 2004

Kharrazian, Datis; *Why Isn't My Brain Working?;* Elephant Press; 2013

Larson, Joan Mathews; *Depression-Free, Naturally: 7 Weeks to Eliminating Anxiety, Despair, Fatigue, and Anger from Your Life;* Wellspring/Bellantine; 2001

May, Jeffery C.; *My House Is Killing Me!: The Home Guide for Families with Allergies and Asthma;* John Hopkins University Press; 2001

Rosen, Gary and Schaller, James; *When Traditional Medicine Fails, Your Guide to Mold Toxins;* Hope Academic Press; 2006

Scott, Trudy; *The Anti-anxiety Food Solution: How the Foods You Eat Can Help You Calm Your Anxious Mind, Improve Your Mood, and End Cravings;* New Harbinger Publication, 2011

Shames, Richard; Shames, Karilee; and Shames, Georjana Grace; *Thyroid Mind Power: The Proven Cure for Hormone-Related Depression, Anxiety, and Memory Loss;* Rodale Books; 2011

Tako, Barbara; *Clutter Clearing Choices: Clear Clutter, Organize Your Home & Reclaim Your Life;* John Hunt Publishing; 2010

Thayer, Robert E.; *Calm Energy: How People Regulate Mood with Food and Exercise;* Oxford University Press; 2003

Turner, Natasha; *The Supercharged Hormone Diet: A 30-Day Accelerated Plan to Lose Weight, Restore Metabolism, and Feel Younger Longer;* Rodale Books; 2013

Vermeulen, Kristy; *Happy Hormones: The Natural Treatment Programs for Weight Loss, PMS, Menopause, Fatigue, Irritability, Osteoporosis, Stress, Anxiety, Thyroid Imbalances and More;* Hatherleigh Press; 2014

About the Author

Michele Pence began her journey with anxiety and treatment options at the tender age of eighteen. After suffering from attention deficit hyperactivity disorder for over twelve years, she experienced her first panic attack. It was a frightening experience to say the least. She had no idea what was happening or what the treatment options were so when her doctor prescribed a daily dose of Xanax, she complied with his treatment recommendations. There was no to know at the time, but it would be a decision she would later fight to overcome.

Never one to remain complacent, she decided to learn more about her condition by earning a degree in Psychology from the University of Central Florida in 2002. There she discovered a passion for helping others. Unfortunately, the sedate world of mental health couldn't hold her. She discovered fast paced profession of sales and marketing were more in line with her true calling. For almost a decade, she has excelled at working with business owners to grow and develop winning marketing campaigns and increase overall sales.

It was her own struggles to better understand the underlying causes of her anxiety that led her to aggressively investigate options for natural health alternatives. She successfully weaned her body off all anxiety medication and sought training as a certified health coach to assist others with their struggles. In 2014, she earned certification as a Certified Health Coach and Board Certified Holistic Health Practitioner through the Institute of Integration Nutrition and the

American Association of Drugless Practitioners as a Holistic Health Healer.

Michele believes that everyone can lead a healthy and productive life with the right lifestyle changes. And she practices what she preaches. An avid exercise enthusiast, she has competed in numerous body building competitions around the country. She is an expert in physical fitness and dietary requirements to enhance your lifestyle challenges and works with people worldwide as they improve their health and bodies.

For more information about Michele and improving your life without medication, contact her for a FREE consultation at www.mindbodyhealthmatters.com/contact. You may also follow her and receive free regular updates by connecting through Twitter (@michelepence) or on Facebook at www.facebook.com/mindbodyhealthmatters. She is available for worldwide consultations through Skype.

Ten percent (10%) of all proceeds from this book will go toward the church and serving the Kingdom of God.

Thank you for reading!!

Dear Reader,

I hope you enjoyed **Find the Root Cause of YOUR Anxiety.** When I first set out on this journey, I had no idea where the road would lead. It was difficult and painful at times, yet I knew I wanted to become a better person not only for myself but also for my family and all those around me. In the end, it became a defining moment in my life. I knew beyond any shadow of a doubt that I had to share my experience with others to hopefully ease their burden.

You, the reader, are the reason this book exists today. And it is my sincerest hope that this book has helped you on your personal journey in some small way. You mean so much to me and I would love to hear your story. You can contact me directly through my website at www.mindbodyhealthmatters.com/contact. Your experience is important to me and if I can be of any help in the future, please do not hesitate to get in touch.

I'd also like to ask you for a favor if you have a spare moment. I'd greatly appreciate your review of the book on either Amazon.com or Goodreads.com. As I'm sure you know, the publishing world has changed drastically over the past few years. Your review is critical in helping others find this book. Whether you loved it, hated it, or somewhere I between, I'd love your feedback and others who are struggling with similar problems would appreciate your help in finding a solution to their battle with anxiety.

Thank you so much for joining me on this journey. I know together, we can alleviate much of the pain of anxiety naturally.

Kindest regards,

Michele Pence

www.ingramcontent.com/pod-product-compliance
Lightning Source LLC
Chambersburg PA
CBHW051654170526
45167CB00001B/460